THE SPRING OF TIMES: A HANBOOK FOR A LONG AND VIBRANT LIFE

By Melton Gatsby

Contents

Chapter 1 - The Pursuit for Longevity and Well-being

The longing for an extended and thriving life is a desire deeply rooted within our human nature. It arises from a sophisticated interplay of fears and vagueness that accompany the passage of time. We contend with the anxiety of observing the gradual decline of our physical vitality and intellectual acuity, as the persistent march of years leaves its permanent mark. The presence of losing the youthful appeal that once defined us emerges like a shadow, a reminder of our mortality.

In this relentless pursuit of longevity, we are, in truth, grappling with the enigma of mortality itself. The inevitability of death, an immutable truth that surrounds us daily, stands as an ever-present sentinel. Yet, despite our cognisance of this reality, embracing the notion that one day we will be reduced to ashes, our corporeal existence transformed into ethereal remnants, remains a formidable challenge.

In confronting our own mortality, we are further entangled in the intricate web of ageing, a journey characterised by its uncertainties and emotional nuances. The prospect of growing old, while a privilege denied to many, carries its own weight of concerns. The anxiety of navigating the twilight years, marked by the erosion of physical prowess and the encroachment of time upon our faculties, adds yet another layer to the complexity of our human experience.

Thus, as we embark on this contemplative expedition, we delve into the profound tapestry of human existence, woven with the threads of hope, trepidation, and resilience. Together, we shall traverse the landscape of longevity, dissecting the intricate threads that comprise the fabric of our aspirations, our apprehensions, and our ceaseless endeavour to not just extend the chronicles of our lives, but to infuse them with purpose, vitality, and enduring significance.

There are many reasons for desiring to live long and healthy. Our motivations will differ from person to person. Many of us want to spend more time with our loved ones, our children, husbands, wives, grandchildren, and even our extended families, boyfriends, or girlfriends. We dearly value the opportunity to deepen and strengthen relationships, create everlasting memories, and support our family members as much as we can for as long as possible.

Embracing a life of enduring prosperity bestows upon us the privilege to savour and relish optimal health and boundless vitality over an extended span. Our aspiration is to safeguard our physical well-being, liberating it from the constraints of persistent maladies, infirmities, or incapacities. Through the gift of longevity, we are presented with the promise of partaking in a superior existence, empowered to engage wholeheartedly in the pursuits and passions that ignite our souls.

The gift of a long life bestows upon us the precious capacity to treasure connections that infuse our days with delight and a profound sense of fulfilment. Amidst the journey of ageing, countless souls aspire to safeguard their self-reliance and sovereignty, a desire to perpetuate the ability to nurture themselves, steer their destinies with autonomy, and embrace existence on their own unique terms.

The value placed upon the opportunity to nurture and fortify relationships with kin, comrades, and cherished individuals extends across the expanse of time. This desire encompasses the intent to cultivate deep-seated bonds and luxuriate in the enduring embrace of these connections woven throughout life's tapestry. For some, the richness of longevity intertwines with the prospect of bearing witness to the unfurling narratives of successive generations, the heirs of their lineage, be it children, grandchildren, or even the distant echo of great-grandchildren.

The human spirit yearns to weave threads of positive contribution into the fabric of its familial legacy, cultivating enduring connections that traverse generations. The heart's ambition seeks not only to imprint a benevolent mark upon the world but to etch it indelibly, a testament to the lasting influence we yearn to bestow.

The canvas of longevity unfurls a vast tableau, where we continue to wield influence, leaving behind footprints of legacy that bridge the span of time. A life well-lived, extended across the years, accumulates a treasury of wisdom, a gallery of adventures, and a trove of lessons culled from the crucible of experience.

The human desire to impart a reservoir of wisdom, skills, expertise, and insights to those who will come after is an enduring yearning. This mentorship, this passing of the torch, stands as a testament to the legacy of knowledge being upheld and perpetuated. The vista of a lengthy life unfurls pathways to chase dreams, cradle ambitions, and harvest personal aspirations. It offers the gift of time, an extended tapestry within which we can diligently pursue the fulfilment of our visions.

These ambitions, as diverse as constellations, may beckon us to master new crafts, talents, or traverse the globe to weave memories through travel's embrace. Others may be drawn to etch an indelible imprint upon the world's canvas, their desire echoing across time. The cadence of longevity harmonises with the symphony of continuous intellectual growth, offering an unfurling print for the strokes of exploration.

Within the expanse of a lengthened existence, individuals continue to harness their thirst for knowledge, fuel their quest for skill enhancement, and remain steadfast in their pursuit of intellectual heights. In this continuum, they forge ahead, walking hand in hand with the spirit of learning, inscribing their story with the ink of everlasting curiosity.

The apprehension of potentially forfeiting forthcoming encounters, revelations, moments of elation, connections, and progressions can act as a rudder, propelling individuals to quest after an extended lifespan. Within this quest resides a yearning to sidestep the shadow of regret, one cast by the inability to bear witness to, or actively participate in future events and breakthroughs.

For those haunted by an unease concerning mortality, the aspiration for an elongated existence assumes the mantle of a countermeasure. The longing for a prolonged life serves as a resolute step toward alleviating the spectre of mortality, offering a sanctuary from the unease. This quest is imbued with the hope that a protracted life might afford the luxury of time, permitting the gradual reconciliation with the concept of finality. This temporal extension, in turn, holds the promise of an enriched voyage toward uncovering spiritual insights, a contemplative exploration to cultivate a more profound understanding of the ineffable mysteries that lie beyond.

The allure of existence holds the potential to kindle a profound longing for an extended life. Within the human spirit resides an ache to bear witness to the evolving narrative of the world, scientific evolution, the cadence of cultural transformations, and the unfurling of fresh revelations.

Emanating from the depths of this sentiment is a potent desire, one that hungers to partake in the symphony of experiences, to bask in the radiance of joys that punctuate life's journey, and to stand in awe of the myriad wonders strewn along its path. This unquenchable thirst, forged from an appreciation for life's exquisite offerings, takes root and propels the heart's steadfast aspiration for an extended life.

A myriad of souls bears within them the weight of unfulfilled aspirations, the echoes of paths untaken and experiences yet to be woven into their stories. It is our unfulfilled desires that ignites the fervent wish for an extended existence, a life generously bestowed with time to chase those longings, to seal the chapters left ajar, and to banish the shadows of regrets.

Rooted deep within the human spirit lies an innate curiosity, a force that propels the heart's compass toward the uncharted territories of existence. This quest, born of an affinity for life's multifaceted wonders, beckons us to traverse new realms, to unearth civilisations that lie veiled in the folds of time, and to drink from the wellspring of novel experiences. In these endeavours, we unearth not just mere interactions, but a trove of joy and contentment, etching our journey with the richness that life's expansive banquet has to offer.

Embracing a prolonged journey enables us the privilege of gazing upon the intricate woven of wildlife, art, music, and the myriad hues of human encounters. It bestows upon us the rare treasure of savouring life's marvels, of becoming not just passive observers, but active participants in the sonata of astonishments that unfold.

Amidst the contours of existence, myriad souls aspire to embrace a retirement marked by unbridled joy, a phase of life where leisure, hobbies, explorations, and cherished moments with kindred spirits takes centre stage. This life stage is envisioned as an orchestration of experiences that harmonise with the heart's desires.

As we tread the path in search of elongated days, there exists a silent hope, a quiet expectation that time's march can be gentled, the effects of ageing softened. The aim is to safeguard the reservoir of freedom and the flame of vitality, allowing us to remain architects of our journeys, both resolute and vibrant.

While the aspiration for a lengthy and flourishing life is a common thread, the landscape of human sentiment is intricate and varied. Indeed, numerous factors can shape an individual's stance on the prospect of longevity. In the presence of relentless health challenges or enduring ailments that cast a shadow over our daily physical abilities and overall wellness, the allure of an extended existence may become a subject of contemplation. The ceaseless weight of these afflictions prompts us to scrutinise the very essence of a prolonged life.

Enduring unyielding pain, limitations, or a perceptible erosion of life's vibrancy can engender a profound cocktail of emotions, frustration, a sense of futility, and an enveloping weariness. Under these taxing circumstances, a yearning may emerge, a gentle yearning for a life that is succinct, unburdened by the shackles of pain and the weight of suffering.

The toll of loss, of beloved ones, cherished family, dear friends, or the companionship of a spouse, casts a poignant hue upon our emotional and social well-being. It leaves an indelible mark, echoing in the corridors of the heart and weaving intricate patterns across the canvas of our existence.

In the wake of such heartaches and the solitude they usher in, a cascade of emotions often compels us to ponder over the profound essence and direction of life itself. From the depths of our souls, we grapple with an ache, a profound solitude that seems to stretch beyond the distance. In this crucible of emotions, the prospect of an elongated life bereft of those held dear can appear to be an insurmountable burden, or even a concept too weighty to bear.

Amidst this contemplation, the thought of reunion with those cherished souls who have departed casts a luminous glow. This ethereal yearning, the whispered hope of embracing loved ones once more in the realm beyond, may cast a shadow upon the desire for a lengthened earthly sojourn. In this narrative of longing, the aspirations for an extended existence take on new dimensions, shimmering against the backdrop of eternal reunions.

The gift of a long life bestows upon us the precious capacity to treasure connections that infuse our days with delight and a profound sense of fulfilment. Amidst the journey of ageing, countless souls aspire to safeguard their self-reliance and sovereignty, a desire to perpetuate the ability to nurture themselves, steer their destinies with autonomy, and embrace existence on their own unique terms.

The value placed upon the opportunity to nurture and fortify relationships with kin, comrades, and cherished individuals extends across the expanse of time. This desire encompasses the intent to cultivate deep-seated bonds and luxuriate in the enduring embrace of these connections woven throughout life's tapestry. For some, the richness of longevity intertwines with the prospect of bearing witness to the unfurling narratives of successive generations, the heirs of their lineage, be it children, grandchildren, or even the distant echo of great-grandchildren.

The human spirit yearns to weave threads of positive contribution into the fabric of its familial legacy, cultivating a tapestry of enduring connections that traverse generations. The heart's ambition seeks not only to imprint a benevolent mark upon the world but to etch it indelibly, a testament to the lasting influence they yearn to bestow.

This noble aspiration takes form as a dedication to buttress communities, society, or a cause that resonates deeply within. Anchored in meaning, this purpose calls for their support, their fervour to empower and uplift. The canvas of longevity unfurls a vast tableau, where they continue to wield their influence, leaving behind footprints of legacy that bridge the span of time. A life well-lived, extended across the tapestry of years, accumulates a treasury of wisdom, a gallery of adventures, and a trove of lessons culled from the crucible of experience.

The human desire to impart their reservoir of wisdom, skills, expertise, and insights to those who will come after is an enduring yearning. This mentorship, this passing of the torch, stands as a testament to the legacy of knowledge being upheld and perpetuated. The vista of a lengthy life unfurls pathways to chase dreams, cradle ambitions, and harvest personal aspirations. It offers the gift of time, an extended tapestry within which they can diligently pursue the fulfilment of their visions.

These ambitions, as diverse as constellations, may beckon them to master new crafts, talents, or traverse the globe to weave memories through travel's embrace. Others may be drawn to etch an indelible imprint upon the world's canvas, their desire echoing across time. The cadence of longevity harmonises with the symphony of continuous intellectual growth, offering an unfurling canvas for the strokes of exploration.

Within the expanse of a lengthened existence, individuals continue to harness their thirst for knowledge, fuel their quest for skill enhancement, and remain steadfast in their pursuit of intellectual heights. In this continuum, they forge ahead, walking hand in hand with the spirit of learning, inscribing their story with the ink of everlasting curiosity.

The apprehension of potentially forfeiting forthcoming encounters, revelations, moments of elation, connections, and progressions can act as a rudder, propelling individuals to quest after an extended lifespan. Within this quest resides a yearning to sidestep the shadow of regret, one cast by the inability to bear witness to, or actively participate in, the tapestry of future events and breakthroughs.

For those haunted by an unease concerning mortality, the aspiration for an elongated existence assumes the mantle of a countermeasure. Through this lens, the longing for a prolonged journey serves as a resolute step toward alleviating the spectre of mortality, offering a sanctuary from the unease. This quest is imbued with the hope that a protracted life might afford the luxury of time, permitting the gradual reconciliation with the concept of finality.

This temporal extension, in turn, holds the promise of an enriched voyage toward uncovering spiritual insights, a contemplative exploration to cultivate a more profound understanding of the ineffable mysteries that lie beyond the horizon.

The allure of existence holds the potential to kindle a profound longing for an extended journey. Within the human spirit resides an ache to bear witness to the evolving narrative of the world, the dance of scientific evolution, the cadence of cultural transformations, and the unfurling of fresh revelations. Nurtured by an abiding and harmonious reverence for the tapestry of existence's splendour, this passion becomes the driving force that fuels the yearning for an elongated sojourn.

Emanating from the depths of this sentiment is a potent desire, one that hungers to partake in the symphony of experiences, to bask in the radiance of joys that punctuate life's journey, and to admire the myriad wonders strewn along its path. This unquenchable thirst, forged from an appreciation for life's exquisite offerings, takes root and propels the heart's steadfast aspiration for an extended voyage.

A myriad of souls bears within them the weight of unfulfilled aspirations, the echoes of paths untaken and experiences yet to be woven into their stories. It is this very tapestry of unfulfilled desires that ignites the fervent wish for an extended existence—a life generously bestowed with time to chase those longings, to seal the chapters left ajar, and to banish the shadows of regrets.

Rooted deep within the human spirit lies an innate curiosity, a force that propels the heart's compass toward the uncharted territories of existence. This quest, born of an affinity for life's multifaceted wonders, beckons us to traverse new realms, to unearth civilisations that lie veiled in the folds of time, and to drink from the wellspring of novel experiences. In these endeavours, we unearth not just mere interactions, but a trove of joy and contentment, etching our journey with the richness that life's expansive banquet has to offer.

Embracing a prolonged journey grants individuals, the privilege of gazing upon the intricate tapestry woven by wildlife, art, music, and the myriad hues of human encounters. It bestows upon them the rare treasure of savouring life's marvels, of becoming not just passive observers, but active participants in the symphony of astonishments that unfold.

Amidst the contours of existence, myriad souls aspire to embrace a retirement marked by unbridled joy, a phase of life where the canvas of leisure, hobbies, explorations, and cherished moments with kindred spirits takes centre stage. This life stage is envisioned as an orchestration of experiences that harmonise with the heart's desires.

As we tread the path in search of elongated days, there exists a silent hope, a quiet expectation that time's march can be gentled, the effects of ageing softened. The aim is to safeguard the reservoir of freedom and the flame of vitality, allowing us to remain architects of our own journey, both resolute and vibrant.

While the aspiration for a lengthy and flourishing life is a common thread, the landscape of human sentiment is intricate and varied. Indeed, numerous factors can shape an individual's stance on the prospect of longevity. In the presence of relentless health challenges or enduring ailments that cast a shadow over their daily physical abilities and overall wellness, the allure of an extended existence may become a subject of contemplation. The ceaseless weight of these afflictions prompts them to scrutinise the very essence of a prolonged life.

Enduring unyielding pain, limitations, or a perceptible erosion of life's vibrancy can engender a profound cocktail of emotions, frustration, a sense of futility, and an enveloping weariness. Under these taxing circumstances, a yearning may emerge, a gentle yearning for a life that is succinct, unburdened by the shackles of pain and the weight of suffering.

The toll of loss of beloved ones, cherished family, dear friends, or the companionship of a spouse, casts a poignant hue upon our emotional and social well-being. It leaves an indelible mark, echoing in the corridors of the heart and weaving intricate patterns across the canvas of our existence.

In the wake of such heartaches and the solitude they usher in, a cascade of emotions often compels individuals to ponder over the profound essence and direction of life itself. From the depths of their souls, they grapple with an ache, a profound solitude that seems to stretch beyond the horizon. In this crucible of emotions, the prospect of an elongated life bereft of those held dear can appear to be an insurmountable burden, or even a concept too weighty to bear.

Amidst this contemplation, the thought of reunion with those cherished souls who have departed casts a luminous glow. This ethereal yearning, the whispered hope of embracing loved ones once more in the realm beyond, may cast a shadow upon the desire for a lengthened earthly sojourn. In this narrative of longing, the aspirations for an extended existence take on new dimensions, shimmering against the backdrop of eternal reunions.

For those grappling with profound mental health struggles, the concept of envisioning a forthcoming chapter, let alone harbouring a desire for an extended lifespan, can prove a formidable task. When confronted with conditions as daunting as severe bipolar disorders, schizophrenia, depression, and anxiety disorders, the intricate interplay between these health challenges and an individual's overall well-being and physical capacities becomes evident.

Within the intricate embroidery of these conditions, emotional anguish stands as a relentless companion, its grip often intertwining with feelings of hopelessness and the pall of despondency. The daunting terrain of mental health struggles can cast a long shadow, one that eclipses the notion of a protracted existence, rendering it a notion that is either unsettling or unwelcome. In these profound chapters of human experience, the notion of seeking a lengthened life may take on hues of complexity, entwined with emotions that are deeply textured and intensely personal.

Certain individuals engage in profound philosophical contemplation, delving into the intricacies of life's essence, the depths of grief, and the enigmatic significance of existence itself. Within these reflective pursuits lies the propensity to unveil inquiries that cast light upon the purpose and significance of a lengthy existence.

Emotions stirred by the transient nature of human beings, the inescapable dance with mortality, or the complexities woven into the fabric of life can kindle a contemplative journey. This introspective odyssey may lead some to raise poignant queries regarding the value of an elongated life. As they grapple with the delicate threads that weave human experiences, these souls embark on a search for resonance and meaning amidst the interplay of life's ephemerality and the enduring echoes of time.

The longing for either an extended or abbreviated lifespan is a nuanced and individualistic pursuit, influenced by a myriad of considerations. Unique life trajectories and external circumstances play a pivotal role in shaping one's aspirations for the duration of existence. For those who experience a fulfilling personal life, profound social ties, robust health, and an overarching sense of purpose, the yearning for an elongated journey may burn brightly. This interwoven fabric of positivity and fulfilment fuels a resolute desire for a longer life, an extension to cherish each moment and continue the intricate waltz with time.

Conversely, those grappling with formidable personal obstacles, enduring health challenges, financial constraints, or a perceptible dimming of life's vibrancy may incline towards an alternate yearning. Their focus may shift from the quantity of days to the quality of those days, prompting an inclination for a more concise journey, a path punctuated by meaningful moments rather than the sheer passage of time.

The role that cultural norms and beliefs assume in shaping individuals' outlooks on the duration of life is of profound significance. Across diverse cultures, the embrace of an extended lifespan can be intricately woven into the fabric of values, aligning itself with notions of wisdom, honour, and social stature. This connection underscores how cultural paradigms can often intertwine with the concept of longevity, painting it with shades of admiration and significance.

Embedded within cultural and religious frameworks lies a powerful influence, one that casts a defining aura over the contours of life and the enigma of mortality. These intricate belief systems become the prism through which individuals perceive the trajectory of existence and the passage into the beyond, contributing to a panorama where the quest for a prolonged life assumes various meanings, enriched by the cultural hues that shape our world.

Within specific cultural settings and age-old traditions, a profound emphasis may be placed on the concept of everlasting life or ethereal domains, where the focus gracefully pivots from the temporal narrative to the eternal and the otherworldly. In these realms, the spotlight shifts, illuminating a path that extends beyond the earthly continuum.

For some, the allure of the journey that unfolds after the mortal coil is shed may eclipse the conventional yearning for a lengthy earthly existence. It is within this cosmic contemplation, shaped by spiritual doctrines and convictions, that perspectives on longevity undergo a transformative reimagining. The desire for a protracted lifespan takes on new contours, cast against the backdrop of spiritual vistas and the tapestries of eternity.

Amidst life's trials and tribulations, there exist those who ardently seek an extended existence, undeterred by the hurdles they encounter. Conversely, there are those who find solace in the present moment, embracing life's organic rhythm of ebbs and flows. Cultural contexts that assign varying significance to the concept of longevity can evoke distinct aspirations among individuals.

At the heart of this variance lie personal convictions, philosophies, and the intricate prism through which life is perceived. These facets of the human experience weave a mosaic of desires for the duration of existence. In essence, the complex interplay of individual beliefs, overarching perspectives, and cultural environments crafts a diverse spectrum of yearnings, shaping the delicate interplay between the yearning for continuity and the embrace of life's transient beauty.

Certain individuals may harbour an ardent longing to traverse the expanse of existence, driven by an unquenchable thirst to immerse themselves in the world's offerings. For them, an extended life stands as a platform upon which personal evolution unfurls its vibrant shades, where aspirations blossom into achievements, and where the very act of being leaves an indelible mark. This perspective crystallises into a fervent desire to shape and be shaped by the world, to engrave a legacy that stands the test of time.

Contrastingly, others find their compass guided by existential or spiritual scopes, charting a course that maps an alternate path. Here, the embrace of life's quality, the intimate communion with the present's tranquillity, and the pursuit of a life imbued with profound significance assume the mantle of precedence. The duration of existence pales in comparison to the luminosity of the moments lived, the depth of contentment experienced, and the echoes of meaning woven into the fabric of their being.

The prism of lived experiences holds within it the power to mould the contours of desires surrounding the duration of existence. Variables including physical well-being, financial security, mental equilibrium, social networks, and the availability of resources all weave threads into the tapestry of aspirations.

For those fortunate enough to traverse the path of robust health, profound connections, financial equilibrium, and experiences of vibrant moments, the call for an extended life is a resonant chord. Nestled within the fabric of their lives are threads of positivity, a mosaic of well-being that invites a yearning to prolong the symphony of life, to allow these cherished experiences to flourish in the boundless expanse of time.

On the other hand, those navigating the maze of enduring pain, emotional turmoil, isolation, or profound distress may voice a predisposition for a briefer journey, a yearning to escape the clutches of suffering. Indeed, affluence can bestow specific privileges and resources that lend us to an enriched existence, adorned with facets such as enhanced quality of life, seamless access to medical aid, and the promise of an extended horizon.

Moreover, the embrace of financial stability can act as a solace, soothing certain strains that might otherwise cast shadows over health and well-being. The absence of financial duress lightens the load on the shoulders of existence, a liberation that fosters an environment more conducive to health, both physical and emotional.

Ultimately, the inclination towards a lengthy existence or otherwise is a multifaceted and deeply personal choice, one that emerges from the intricate interplay of myriad influences.

The intricacies of an individual's views on mortality, as well as their connection with the enigma of death itself, can reverberate profoundly in shaping their aspirations for the duration of life.

For some, a palpable aversion to the notion of death might cast a shadow, compelling a fervent yearning for prolonged days to forestall its inevitable arrival. The prospect of an extended journey becomes a mechanism to hold at bay the certainty of mortality, a chance to grasp a few more fleeting moments before yielding to the enigmatic beyond.

Others may adopt a more embracing or rational vantage point, one that acknowledges the organic rhythm of existence. With an understanding of life's natural order and the cyclical rave it embodies, they come to terms with mortality. This acceptance blends seamlessly with the concept of death and nurturing contentment in the face of the inevitable.

Desires pertaining to life span can vary among individuals. While many individuals express a desire for a prolonged life, it is critical to acknowledge diverse perspectives and individual autonomy in establishing what represents a fulfilling life. In the end, personal values, beliefs, and the quality of life lived impact the complexities of desires surrounding a longer life span.

The aspiration for an extended lifespan yields a plethora of advantages. Individuals endowed with a steadfast determination and a profound sense of life's purpose may find themselves reaping the rewards of enhanced physical well-being and a diminished vulnerability to mortality from diverse sources. The prospect of prolonged longevity holds the potential to embolden individuals to remain active in their professional spheres for extended periods, an endeavour that offers a constellation of merits.

This continued engagement not only nurtures ongoing mental stimulation through work that resonates deeply, but also nurtures an unwavering sense of determination. As a result, it stands as a formidable shield against the encroachment of solitude, serving as a catalyst to thwart its onset. Moreover, an extended work life paves the way for the accumulation of resources over a more expansive temporal canvas, affording ample opportunity to build wealth and leave a lasting imprint.

A probable rise in life expectancy is expected as the years unfold. Lifelong learning is emerging as a magnet, drawing both the youthful and the mature towards the pursuit of elevated educational tiers. This endeavour not only imparts discipline but also serves as a catalyst, urging individuals to chase their aspirations throughout the entire arc of their existence. Moreover, this educational odyssey has the potential to weave a robust connection among individuals who share a common intellectual fervour, spanning a diverse spectrum of society.

Adopting a purpose infused life can become a beacon, illuminating the path towards emotional and physical well-being. It forms a stronghold against the looming spectres of cardiac ailments and other potentially fatal health conditions. The art of embracing a health-conscious lifestyle further amplifies these endeavours. Engaging in regular exercise, adhering to a nourishing diet, and refraining from smoking become pivotal components in the orchestration of physical vitality. This symphony of choices does more than enhance the body's wellness, it also extends the horizons of existence, paving the way for an elongated life.

The bedrock of a prolonged existence lies in well-being, which assumes a pivotal role for a multitude of compelling reasons. Elevated levels of well-being are intricately intertwined with an extended life, a shield against the encroachment of ailments and injuries, while also unfurling the petals of a fortified immune system.

Those who cultivate a sound mental and spiritual equilibrium are naturally inclined towards nurturing their physical health. This nurturing reveals itself through an active lifestyle, sound sleep, and a penchant for preventive health practices that seamlessly intertwine with physical well-being and the promise of an elongated life.

Well-being transcends its domain to blend connections with life satisfaction, overall health, and a profound sense of contentment. This interconnection reverberates through the rhythm of daily life, infusing each moment with the potential to extract more from life. The nurturing of meaningful relationships is an act that fosters not just happiness but also health, it stands as a testament to the symbiotic interplay between connection and longevity.

Enhancing well-being encompasses a myriad of avenues. For numerous individuals, this journey unfolds through the cultivation of positive relationships, where like-minded souls connect and commune. Within this intricate network, the seeds of acceptance and self-value are sown, giving rise to a sanctuary of emotional sustenance. Not only do these connections offer solace and camaraderie, but they also open the wings of altruism, enabling individuals to support one another on the shared voyage of life.

The fabric of well-being is further woven through the threads of gratitude, restful slumber, regular exercise, and adept stress management. Individuals adeptly navigate the ebbs and flows of emotions, adeptly steering through stress, depression, and anxiety. They engage in the art of acquiring new skills, a pursuit that not only enriches their mental landscape but also elevates their reservoirs of confidence. The acquisition of fresh abilities acts as a solace, nurturing mental well-being by igniting self-assuredness and kindling a profound sense of purpose.

Generosity and acts of kindness are also especially important. These gestures birth a symphony of positive emotions, enveloping individuals in the glow of reward and fulfilment. This radiant aura fosters a sanctuary of mental well-being, where the seeds of purpose and self-esteem take root and flourish, painting life's canvas with hues of significance and intrinsic worth.

Mindfulness holds the potential to kindle a profound appreciation for life's intricacies, nurturing a deepened understanding of oneself, and orchestrating a positive metamorphosis in the prism through which life is perceived, reshaping perspectives on existence and the way adversities are navigated.

The practice of mindfulness exercises extends a gentle hand, steering attention away from the clutches of negative ruminations and guiding individuals towards an intimate engagement with the present realm. This voyage births a harmonious resonance, culminating in the alleviation of stress, the dispelling of apprehension, and the softening of the shadows cast by depression.

In the gentle embrace of mindfulness, life's joys are not mere spectacles, but treasures to be savoured. It becomes a vessel to immerse oneself wholeheartedly in each activity, unlocking an elevated capacity to confront the tempestuous waters of life's trials. This resilience kindles a gentle luminosity within, fostering an elevated emotional climate. Ultimately, the art of mindfulness weaves enriched emotional experiences, crafting a sanctuary where life is cherished, presence is paramount, and the journey infused with the tones of a buoyant spirit.

Mindfulness meditation stands as a cornerstone within the realm of treating a myriad of mental health afflictions. From the depths of depression to the clutches of drug abuse, from the turmoil of eating disorders to the grip of anxiety disorders and obsessive-compulsive tendencies, its therapeutic influence has resonated profoundly.

Embedded within mindfulness practices lies the potential to unfurl transformative change. A voyage embarked upon by those who seek a compass for purpose, an elixir for kindling positive emotions, and a balm to nurture flourishing relationships. Even the realms of productivity, inspiration, and altruism find themselves touched by its grace, as workplaces witness heightened dedication, creativity finds new wellsprings of inspiration, and the bloom of prosocial behaviour graces the hearts of people.

The spectrum of mindfulness practices unfolds through a tapestry of meditative rituals, contemplative pursuits, and purposeful engagements. Within this rich tapestry, lies the transformative potential to elevate well-being on myriad fronts. Through the gentle touch of mindfulness, stress relinquishes its grip, apprehensions find solace, and the shadows of depression recede. A harmonious temperament takes root, psychological well-being flourishes, and the journey towards enhanced mental health gains momentum. With each mindful step, personal growth finds fertile ground, paving the way for a holistic blossoming.

Neglecting the quest for well-being unfurls consequential setbacks. Those who veer away from the pursuit of happiness often find themselves ensnared by the tendrils of misery and the burden of suffering. A profound correlation emerges between heightened well-being and the embroidery of beneficial outcomes, particularly in the realm of physical health and the expanse of longevity.

Individuals who stand at the summit of well-being not only cast a radiant glow upon their personal lives but also upon their professional arena. Their footsteps within the workplace resonate with heightened productivity, fuelled by the alchemy of contentment. The quest for knowledge finds a willing partner in their enriched state, as learning becomes a harmonious endeavour. Within the theatre of creativity, their minds take flight, traversing uncharted realms of innovation. And as they navigate the complex landscape of relationships, their journey is adorned with the jewels of positivity and enduring connections.

Overlooking the pursuit of effective treatment for conditions like depression casts a shadow that darkens both mental and physical well-being, while also sowing the seeds of diminished concentration and enduring challenges. In the realm of well-being, those who dwell in its lower echelons find themselves entangled in a web of discontentment and disquiet, their aspirations rendered listless by lacklustre motivation.

The importance of cultivating robust mental health reverberates, for it equips individuals with the fortitude to navigate stress's tempestuous waters. In this realm, the pursuit of well-being stands as an unequivocal imperative, a compass guiding the way toward resilience and equilibrium. By embracing this journey, the toll of toxic physiological responses to stress finds mitigation, casting a luminous glow upon the path to holistic wellness.

Chapter 2 - The Science of Ageing

Gerontology, the scientific exploration of the ageing process, presents itself as a captivating and intricate domain. Within its embrace, a rich mosaic of complexities unravels, shedding light on the sophisticated dimensions and ramifications of advancing years. Through a multidisciplinary lens, gerontology intertwines the cords of biology, psychology, and sociology, embarking on a quest to unveil the enigmas that shroud the mechanisms and motivations underlying the journey of ageing.

In its pursuit, gerontology embarks upon an odyssey that seeks not only to decipher the intricate means or reasons of ageing but also to illuminate the pathways toward enhancing well-being and enriching the fabric of life's later chapters. This field stands as a beacon guiding us through the uncharted waters of our later years, fostering a deeper understanding of the intricate interplay between time's passage and the art of living fully.

In the contemporary landscape, comprehending the intricacies of the science of ageing has risen to paramount significance, an imperative embraced not only by the scientific community but also by society at large. This pressing relevance has been accentuated by the ever-expanding global population.

Gerontology, weaves together a myriad of disciplines into its narrative fabric. Within its scope, the threads of biology, genetics, medicine, psychology, sociology, and public health intersect, forming a mosaic of knowledge. Collaborative efforts among scholars across these diverse domains converge to unravel the mysteries shrouding the mechanisms governing the ageing process. They endeavour to elucidate the catalysts that set age-related transformations in motion, whether in body or mind, while also casting a discerning gaze upon the profound reverberations ageing imparts across the vast spectrum of human existence.

Nestled within the core pursuits of gerontology lies a paramount fascination, the revelation of the elaborate biological underpinnings that orchestrate the symphony of ageing, both on the scale of the organism and within the realm of molecules. Within the hallowed halls of scientific inquiry, topics of profound import, including cellular senescence, the gradual dwindling of telomeres, the intricate interplay of DNA damage, and the weighty influence of oxidative stress upon the ageing narrative, have been meticulously examined.

With a discerning gaze, researchers have delved into the involved corridors of knowledge, seeking to decipher the enigmatic interplay between these factors and the delicate ballet that is ageing. The dynamic interweaving of genetic endowment and the brushstrokes of the environment have been laid bare upon the canvas of inquiry. The tempo at which the curtain falls on youth's stage and the susceptibility to ailments of age converge, creating a panorama of insights that continues to shape the contours of our understanding.

Another cornerstone within the sphere of gerontology rests upon the understanding of the psychological facets intrinsic to the ageing process. This pursuit involves a deep exploration into the complex mosaic of mental metamorphoses, the delicate traces of emotional equilibrium, and the concerto of social interactions at play through the chapters of advancing years.

Gerontology casts a spotlight upon the complex societal implications spun by an ageing population. It explores the intricate relationship between challenges and prospects unfurled by a maturing populace. This all-encompassing quest delves into the profound realms of healthcare demands and the need for sustained long-term care, the workings of retirement intricacies and the art of fiscal preparation, as well as the pressing dialogue around age-based biases and the delicate opus of intergenerational bonds.

In its pursuit, gerontology exposes an involved mosaic that captures the essence of age within society, unearthing the profound dynamics at play. It elucidates the dimensions of human experience in these later chapters of life, revealing the paths that lead towards holistic well-being through a framework of solidarity and support.

By understanding the science of ageing, we can carefully encourage an innate appreciation for the fullness and multiplicity of the ageing process and oeuvre towards building a society that appreciates and supports individuals across their entire lifespan. Understanding the ageing process helps us improve tactics and involvements geared towards advance healthy ageing.

Through diligent study, we can unlock the ability to decode the complex biological, psychological, and societal forces that orchestrate the rhythm of age-related transformations. Armed with these insights, a realm of possibilities exists, preventive strategies spring forth, lifestyles metamorphose, and tailored interventions take shape. The fruits of these efforts harvest an enriched landscape of physical and mental vitality as we traverse the later stages of life.

Fundamental to this narrative is the profound understanding that age stands as a key player, a pivot upon which numerous health destinies hinge. It is the swivel upon which risks take form, shaping the journey toward afflictions like cardiac anomalies, cancer's stealthy advance, the invasions of neurodegenerative disorders, and the shadow of diabetes.

Through the acquisition of insights into the mechanisms underpinning the journey of ageing, we glean a philosophical understanding of the niceties at the atomic and microscopic levels that fuel age-related maladies. This comprehension emerges as a hub for the progression of impactful diagnostic instruments, transformative interventions aimed at restoration, and the arrangement of strategies for the adept management of age-related diseases.

The process of ageing ushers in an array of challenges and transformations, encompassing realms both physical and psychological. By navigating these shifts with understanding, the door opens to crafting interventions that stand as fortifications against the erosion of age-related decline. These interventions, bearing the potential to elevate life in one's later years, cast a wide net.

They embrace the fostering of mental equilibrium, the preservation of mobility's grace, the nurturing of cognitive vitality, and the cultivation of connections that transcend the social fabric. In this orchestra of care, the golden chapters of life may be lived with enriched resonance and enduring vibrancy.

As comprehension dawns upon individuals regarding the journey of ageing, the curtain of conventional misconceptions and stereotypical notions surrounding the elder years is poised to lift. This enlightenment becomes a forerunner of a discerning and polished comprehension, one that unveils the collage of diversity and potentials embedded within aged individuals.

Yet, in the face of these revelations, the phantom of ageism remains. A challenge beckons to confront and disband this forerunner of bias. By embarking upon this journey, societies carve a path that ushers in attitudes of positivity towards the unfolding years. Through this transformation, the seeds of inclusivity take root, while the bloom of respect for the elder generation flourishes, weaving a fabric that interlaces the threads of wisdom, experience, and collective humanity.

The elaborate journey of ageing encompasses a complicated interplay of multifarious elements, operating seamlessly at both the cellular and molecular realms of existence. While the exact mechanisms continue to unfold within the space of research and understanding, several pivotal pathways have emerged, etching their significance into the montage of the ageing process.

Among the sonata of biological phenomena entwined with ageing, there stand out prominent players like cellular senescence, the waning of telomeres, the scars of DNA damage, the shifting landscapes of epigenetic modifications, the vacillating cadence of mitochondria, the delicate balance of protein equilibrium, the ember of inflammation, and the metamorphosis of hormonal orchestration.

Telomeres, those vigilant sentinels gracing the termini of chromosomes, embark on a gradual diminuendo with every cell division they oversee. This orchestrated attenuation of telomeres stands as an emblem of the ageing narrative. As these chromosomal custodians find themselves notably abbreviated, the cells they safeguard embark on a fateful crossroads, veering towards the path of replicative senescence or programmed cellular oblivion. In this intricate waltz, tissues, and organs, once orchestrated in harmonious function, falter and wane.

Telomeres assume a pivotal role in the orchestration of cellular ageing and the preservation of genetic integrity. In each instance of cellular division, DNA replication processes encounter a limitation, it falters at the culmination of chromosomes, unable to fully replicate their extremities. Thus, the once dignified telomeres embark on a gradual procession of reduction with each successive cell division. Yet, in the crescendo of this biological sonnet, a poignant reckoning awaits. When these guardians of the chromosomal orbit find themselves perilously abbreviated, they incite a cellular overture, an elegy of programmed demise.

This intricate mechanism serves as a defence against the generation of cells bearing flawed or precarious genetic information, thereby playing a pivotal role in the receding of tissue efficacy and the advent of maladies tethered to the passage of time. With the march of years, senescent cells accrue, stealthily releasing a cascade of molecules that stir the flames of inflammation and unleash a torrent of ruinous agents, culminating in the endurance of prolonged inflammation and the consequent compromise of tissue integrity.

Over the expanse of time, the very essence of DNA succumbs to an array of impairments, a result of an intricate interplay between internal forces and the ceaseless barrage of external elements, the harrowing caress of oxidative onslaught, radiation, and the entanglement with noxious elements cast adrift in the environment.

The convoluted intricacies of ageing and the ailments entwined with advancing years find a nexus in the flawed workings of DNA repair mechanisms, coupled with the gradual accrual of genetic lesions. With the rise of cellular senescence, cells embrace a perpetual stasis, a cessation of their once ceaseless division and replication.

The gradual compilation of mutations in the mitochondrial DNA, a diminishment of mitochondrial vigour, and the crescendo of oxidative tension orchestrate a masterpiece of changes. Over the annals of time, the scales tip towards a dissonant pulse, an imbalance in cellular vitality and a progressive attenuation of cellular efficacy, casting a sober narrative upon the unfolding chronicles of ageing.

Proteins assume a precarious role in coordinating cellular function and upholding overall cellular well-being. As the years advance, complexities may arise in the synthesis, folding, and degradation of proteins, culminating in the accumulation of impaired protein structures. This sophisticated interplay can disturb the delicate equilibrium of cellular harmony, consequently fostering the emergence of age-associated maladies.

Concurrently, a chronic state of low-grade inflammation, often referred to as "inflammaging," emerges as a hallmark of the ageing process. This phenomenon is characterised by an upsurge in pro-inflammatory agents juxtaposed with a decline in the presence of anti-inflammatory factors.

The cyclical presence of inflammation bears the weight of inflicting harm upon delicate tissues, undermining the functionality of vital organs, and inadvertently fostering the onset of ailments affiliated with the passing of time. As years advance, the ebb and flow of hormonal equilibrium come to the forefront.

The gradual decline in growth hormones, the subtle wane in sex hormones like oestrogen and testosterone, and the slight shift in insulin-like growth factor-1 (IGF-1) intricately weave themselves into the fabric of the ageing narrative, exerting influence over multifarious aspects of cellular operation and the complex upkeep of bodily tissues.

Mitochondrial dysfunction encapsulates the abnormal functioning of mitochondria, which are the cellular organelles needed to generate energy in the form of adenosine triphosphate (ATP), through the intricate process of cellular respiration. Mitochondria assume a significant role in numerous cellular mechanisms, including calcium homeostasis, reactive oxygen species (ROS) regulation, and apoptosis (programmed cell death).

A myriad of factors facilitates the onset of mitochondrial dysfunction. Inherited mutations within mitochondrial DNA (mtDNA) or nuclear genes, responsible for encoding mitochondrial proteins, hold the potential to disrupt the innate architecture and operation of mitochondria. These genetic deviations wield influence over a multitude of facets tied to mitochondrial function, spanning from the production of adenosine triphosphate (ATP) to the activity of the electron transport chain and the generation of reactive oxygen species (ROS).

Mitochondria embody a dual role as both generators and recipients of reactive oxygen species (ROS), inevitable by-products of the cellular respiration process. When the production of ROS exceeds reasonable levels, or the defensive capabilities of antioxidants fall short, oxidative stress ensues.

This stress detrimentally affects the components within mitochondria, imposing hindrances upon their operational prowess. Noteworthy is the fact that mitochondria undergo an array of dynamic processes, among them fusion, a convergence of mitochondria, and fission, a partitioning of mitochondria. Trepidations in these intricate processes can herald remodelled mitochondrial shapes and compromised functionality.

Exposure to environmental toxins such as heavy metals, pesticides, and certain drugs, can meddle with mitochondrial function. Factors like chronic swelling, nutrient deficiencies, and metabolic conditions can also affect mitochondrial dysfunction. The consequences of mitochondrial dysfunction can be far reaching because mitochondria are critical for the suitable functioning of practically all cell types.

The decline in adenosine triphosphate (ATP) synthesis culminates in a decrease in cellular energy reserves, consequently triggering sensations of weariness, muscular debilitation, and a decline in overall physical prowess. Organs and tissues that exhibit elevated energy requisites such as the brain, heart, and muscles, remain particularly susceptible to the ramifications of mitochondrial disruption. The malfunctioning of mitochondria yields an amplification in the production of reactive oxygen species (ROS), fostering oxidative harm to essential cellular constituents including proteins, lipids, and DNA.

The repercussions of this oxidative stress extend to a spectrum of afflictions, including neurodegenerative disorders, cardiovascular maladies, and even cancer. The disruption in mitochondrial function can thornily disturb the equilibrium of regular metabolism, subsequently ending in metabolic anomalies, including insulin resistance, obesity, and dyslipidaemia.

In this complicated interplay, mitochondrial dysfunction assumes culpability for an array of conditions, ranging from mitochondrial disorders and neurodegenerative diseases to cardiovascular ailments, metabolic disruptions, and the inevitable decline that accompanies the passage of time.

Assuming a pivotal function, mitochondrial dysfunction orchestrates the intricate symphony of programmed cell death, commonly recognised as apoptosis. Within this orchestration, it discharges an array of molecules, most notably cytochrome c, which in turn instigates the activation of caspases, an ensemble of proteins dedicated to inaugurating the complex cascade of apoptosis. This intricately choreographed procedure harmonises the elimination of cells marred by damage or redundancy, serving as the foundation for developmental refinement, tissue restructuring, and the orchestration of immune responses.

Embedded within the narrative of cellular dynamics is the accumulation of oxidative damage inflicted by free radicals, a central protagonist in the ageing narrative. These free radicals, characterised by their reactivity and unpaired electrons, traverse a capricious trajectory, often resulting in the impairment of essential cellular components, encompassing proteins, lipids, and the intricate DNA tapestry.

Accumulating gradually with the passage of time, this damage assumes a cumulative role in composing the persistent degradation of cellular functionality, thereby actively contributing to the intricate process of ageing.

Cultivating a wellness-centric lifestyle, underscored by a well-balanced diet replete with antioxidants, coupled with consistent physical engagement, and a conscious avoidance of undue encounters with environmental pollutants, collectively align to mitigate the impact of oxidative harm. Such conscientious efforts pave the way for a sustained defence against cellular decline and fosters the prospect of a flourishing journey into the realm of healthy ageing.

In the elaborate sphere of genetics, the term "genomic instability" emerges as a profound concept, encapsulating the genome's inherent propensity for metamorphosis and mutation. This proclivity, while a cornerstone of evolution, can also unveil a disquieting facet, a fragility that disrupts the very essence of genetic authenticity and equilibrium.

Genomic instability often portends an underlying narrative of diseases and ailments. It serves as a harbinger of genetic disarray. Intriguingly, amid the shadowy contours of genomic instability, lies a complex alliance with the inexorable march of time, the ageing process. Like a ragged script, the genome accumulates notations and errata, each change, a footnote in the story of life's passage. The symposium between genomic instability and ageing is as complex as it is profound, an eternal waltz etched by the expert choreographers of genetics, environment, and cellular dynamics.

Genomic instability is not a colossal force but rather a multifaceted phenomenon sculpted by the deft interplay of myriad elements. Genetic strands, interconnected through generations, play their part, environmental mutters echo in its chambers, and the ceaseless recital of cellular processes leaves its imprints. This convergence births a sonata of changes, a complex composition spun from the threads of variability.

In the grand scheme of things, genomic instability takes centre stage, both as a creator and a disruptor. Its narrative, sophisticated and compelling, is a testament to the boundless complexities that underscore the living code of existence. It beckons us to delve deeper, to explore the delicate equilibrium that balances change and stability, evolution, and fragility, in the eternal journey of the genome.

It plays a pivotal role in fostering genetic modifications, with profound implications for the commencement and advancement of tumours, frequently culminating in the genesis of malignant cells. In the sophisticated process of DNA replication, errors may transpire, giving rise to substitutions, insertions, or even omissions of nucleotides within the genetic sequence.

These replication anomalies can be ascribed to aberrations within DNA repair mechanisms or deficiencies in the DNA itself. Such aberrations are often elicited by an array of factors, including exposure to radiation and specific chemicals. Consequently, this detriment to DNA integrity can precipitate fractures in the DNA strands, interconnections between them, or chemical modifications to the foundational DNA bases.

Within the cellular space, complex DNA repair machinery operates with a precision that identifies and rectifies instances of DNA damage. Yet, when deficiencies or mutations afflict DNA repair genes, the repair process itself encounters hindrances, allowing for the accrual of

DNA lesions. This, in turn, escalates the susceptibility to genomic instability. Such instability can trigger mutations, enduring alterations in the DNA sequence that imprint their mark.

Mutations wield the power to sway the customary operations of genes, casting their impact upon protein synthesis, the coordination of cellular proliferation, and an array of other intricate molecular endeavours. Their repercussions can extend to a significant overhaul of chromosomal architecture, subsequently setting the stage for genetic syntheses, the amplification of pivotal genes, or the lamentable vanishing act of tumour suppressor genes. This complex interplay ultimately heralds the onset of cancer's insidious evolution.

Stem cell depletion alludes to the decline in the regenerative prowess and operational capacity of stem cells, manifesting under specific circumstances or because of advancing age. Stem cells, those remarkable undifferentiated entities, possess the unparalleled dual capability of self-renewal and the transformative journey towards becoming distinct cell lineages. Their composition assumes a paramount role in orchestrating the repair, rejuvenation, and perpetual upkeep of bodily tissues across the entire spectrum of an individual's existence.

Stem cells undertake the vital task of rejuvenating and mending weathered or senescent tissues, serving as a fresh battalion of cells poised to supplant the ranks of the compromised or expiring ones. These versatile entities are distributed within various bodily tissues and organs, notably including the marrow of bones, the integumentary shelter of skin, the complex recesses of the cerebral domain, and the sinews that empower muscles.

Yet, as the sands of time sift or the unfurling embroidery of chronic ailments unravels, the functional heroism of stem cells may falter, succumbing to a gradual dimming. Through the voyage of existence, they confront a persistent bombardment from agents that scathe the integrity of their DNA, as well as the relentless ravages of oxidative turmoil. This perpetual exposure sketches a portrait of DNA damage and genetic mutations that can accumulate surreptitiously, casting shadows upon the once-promising legacy of stem cells.

The diminished efficacy of DNA repair mechanisms within aged stem cells stands as a significant catalyst for the emergence of genomic instability and the ensuing wane in functional aptitude. The cradle of stem cell activity, known as the stem cell niche, occupies a pivotal function in the orchestration of stem cell performance.

Yet, the passing of time or the encroachments of maladies can coordinate shifts within this specialised microenvironment, exacting a toll upon the flourishing of stem cells. In particular, the spectre of chronic inflammation casts its shadow upon the vitality of stem cells, potentially ushering them towards the precipice of exhaustion. This ominous progression bears consequential implications for tissue repair and the rekindling of regenerative potential.

The waning regenerative prowess exhibited by fatigued stem cells bears consequences of considerable gravity, a diminished capacity for tissue repair, heightened vulnerability to injury, and a gradual decline in organ vitality. The comprehension of the complex mechanisms underpinning the phenomenon of stem cell exhaustion assumes paramount importance, as it holds the key to devising strategies that can rejuvenate these cellular sentinels and promote graceful ageing.

Diligent researchers are ardently delving into a repertoire of innovative methodologies. Among these, there exists the tantalising prospect of rejuvenating aged stem cells, coaxing them back to a state of youthful vigour. Another avenue of inquiry involves the manipulation of the stem cell niche, the microenvironment in which these remarkable cells reside, in the hopes of rekindling their regenerative potential. The realm of stem cell-based therapies beckons, offering the exciting possibility of mitigating or forestalling the inexorable march of stem cell exhaustion, thereby enhancing tissue regeneration, and hindering the inevitable progress of ageing.

Hormone Replacement Therapy, abbreviated as HRT, serves as a remedy for the waning levels of hormones within the body. Its essence lies in the art of elevating these vital messengers to a state reminiscent of youth. As a pertinent example, when it comes to postmenopausal women, the judicious application of hormone replacement therapy, which includes the likes of oestrogen and progesterone, not only serves to alleviate troublesome symptoms but also curbs the peril posed by certain age-related maladies.

However, it is of paramount importance to bear in mind that the advantages and potential pitfalls of embarking on this therapeutic path can be a nuanced affair, with outcomes contingent upon individual factors, demanding the utmost diligence in contemplation.

In the sphere of genetic science, methods like genetic engineering have opened intriguing avenues for the modulation of the ageing process. Within this intriguing field, scientists have uncovered the intricate web of genes and genetic pathways that exert profound influence over the lifespan and overall well-being of model organisms. By deftly manipulating these genetic levers, there arises an exciting possibility, the augmentation of lifespan and the deferment of age-related afflictions.

Yet, the journey doesn't end here. A burgeoning area of exploration involves the precise targeting and elimination of senescent cells through the application of senolytic drugs or innovative strategies. These pioneering endeavours have not merely hinted at potential, they have, in fact, yielded compelling results. In animal studies, the promise is undeniable, marked enhancements in health and a protracted existence have become tangible possibilities.

Caloric restriction, or CR, stands as a nutritional strategy that artfully treads the line of curbing calorie consumption without veering into malnutrition's perilous territory. It entails the art of consuming fewer calories than the daily norm, all while safeguarding the essential nourishment required for well-being. This disciplined approach to dietary restraint has consistently unfurled its remarkable potential, bestowing the gift of extended life across species.

In the sphere of scientific inquiry, an array of studies has unfolded, revealing the significant impact of caloric restriction on longevity. In these investigations, it becomes evident that animals subjected to this regimen traverse the sands of time, outlasting their counterparts on conventional diets. The precise magnitude of this lifespan expansion, however, waltzes to its own tune, swaying to the genetic harmonies of each species, and the caloric restriction regimen applied.

Caloric restriction, far from being a one-dimensional marvel, not only helps extend lifespan but also paints it with vibrant hues of health and vitality. This encompasses what we term the "health span", a phase of existence defined by the twin blessings of robust health and functional prowess.

Beneath the regimen of caloric restraint, subjects often unveil a captivating narrative of resilience against the onslaught of time. They emerge as protagonists of a tale where age-related maladies, from the spectre of cardiovascular disease to the shadow of cancer, from neurodegenerative disorders to the burdens of metabolic ailments, are not only delayed but also softened in their ferocity.

The practice of caloric restriction unfurls a symphony of metabolic transformations within the body's intricate framework. It orchestrates a ballet of adaptations, including heightened insulin sensitivity, refined glucose regulation, diminished blood pressure, attenuated inflammation, and a reconfiguration of lipid metabolism.

These intricate enzymatic shifts, akin to the tuning of instruments in an orchestra, underpin the tapestry of health benefits that grace the realm of caloric restriction. This disciplined dietary approach sets in motion a harmonious interplay of cellular stress responses and the activation of nutrient-sensing pathways. These pathways, like diligent custodians, oversee the absorption of energy, bolster resilience against stress, and orchestrate the meticulous maintenance of cellular integrity.

Caloric restriction emerges as a potent ally in the relentless battle against oxidative stress. This enigmatic adversary, characterised by an imbalance between the production of reactive oxygen species (ROS) and the fortifications of the antioxidant defence system, finds its equilibrium disrupted.

Within the arena of caloric restraint, a subtle yet profound transformation unfolds. As calorie intake dwindles, the incendiary production of reactive oxygen species, arising from the crucible of metabolic processes, is gently subdued. This measured reduction acts as a shield, a guardian of sorts, fortifying cells and tissues against the ravages of oxidative damage.

In the intricate work of biological rejuvenation, caloric restriction assumes the role of a custodian, diligently preserving the vital function of stem cells. These enigmatic agents of regeneration hold the keys to tissue repair, ensuring the ongoing melody of vitality. However, it is a delicate dance, one that demands a discerning balance.

Prolonged caloric restriction, when pursued without due regard for adequate nutrition, can unfurl a discordant tune. The consequences, though not immediate, may manifest as the mournful notes of malnutrition, the gradual erosion of muscle mass, the dissonance of hormonal imbalances, and other adverse effects.

Individual responses to caloric restriction may vary from person to person. Each of us, akin to a soloist, may exhibit variations and fine points in response to this regimen. Thus, the tale of caloric restriction is a narrative both compelling and diverse, that elusive balance between restriction and sustenance is so critical.

Exercise, the artful orchestration of physical movement, choreographs a symphony within the human form. With each deliberate step and motion, it commands an ascent in energy expenditure, crafting a pathway toward the coveted caloric deficit. This discipline, however, transcends mere calorie balance, it emerges as a steadfast pillar underpinning the edifice of holistic health and well-being.

In the domain of our well-being, the merits of regular exercise ripple across the physical, mental, and emotional realms. It bestows upon the heart a mantle of resilience, fine-tuning its rhythm to a harmonious beat. Blood, guided by this rhythm, flows with newfound vitality, a lifeline that reduces the ominous spectre of cardiovascular ailments. Exercise is not just a physical endeavour but a masterpiece that paints vibrant strokes across the canvas of our existence, enriching our lives in myriad ways.

Exercise, akin to a well-tuned instrument, plays a multifaceted tune within the grand symphony of health. With each purposeful movement, it acts as the virtuoso conductor orchestrating a harmonious balance. This rhythmic endeavour is a furnace for calories, a sculptor of weight management, an alchemist of metabolism. It forges the sinew of muscle, cultivating strength and endurance, while modelling flexibility and performance into a seamless composition.

Beyond the stage of physicality, exercise becomes a guardian of longevity. It fine-tunes the body's machinery, enhancing insulin sensitivity, regulating glucose, and harmonising lipid profiles, thereby lowering the curtains on the looming menaces of diabetes and metabolic disorders.

Even in its most moderate manifestations, exercise emerges as a guardian of our well-being, nurturing the immune system's resilience and erecting fortifications against infection and illness. Its magic touch conjures forth endorphins, those enchanting "feel-good" elixirs of the brain, ushering in a brighter mood while gently dissipating stress, depression, and anxiety.

Yet, exercise is not content with bestowing these emotional benedictions alone. It extends its embrace to the realm of cognition, fostering sharper faculties of memory, attention, and physical prowess. With each stride, it whispers to the body, coaxing stress levels to subside, orchestrating a serene ballet of cortisol reduction and the symphonic rise of neurotransmitters like serotonin and dopamine. Exercise reveals itself as a multifaceted gem of health and vitality, each facet catching the light of well-being from a different angle.

In the dominion of rest, exercise emerges as a trusted ally, nurturing the tranquillity of slumber with both quality and quantity. It weaves a tapestry of improved sleep patterns, inviting the embrace of restorative rest. Yet, its benefits are not confined to the nocturnal hours alone. Regular exercise stands as a guardian against the looming threats of chronic ailments. In its vigilant company, cardiovascular diseases, diabetes, cancer, hypertension, arthritis, and the persistent ache of chronic pain find their threats diminished.

Beyond the horizon of immediate health, the consistent rhythm of physical activity extends its promises. It is the orchestrator of an extended lifespan and the quiet conductor of reduced mortality rates. In this masterpiece of well-being, exercise remains the steadfast composer of a harmonious and enduring melody.

Exercise assumes a leading role in the delicate art of preserving our autonomy, safeguarding the fortitude of muscle, and fending off age-related wear and tear, both in body and mind. It is a guardian of functional independence, a vigilant custodian of strength, and a shield against the withering tides of cognitive decline.

In the world of physical activity, a rich tapestry of exercises unfolds, each playing its distinctive role in nurturing well-being. The brisk footsteps of walking, the soaring strides of running, the graceful strokes of swimming, the relentless revolutions of cycling, and the vibrant rhythms of dance all come together on a shared stage, harmonising in a symphony that elevates cardiovascular fitness. But the repertoire doesn't end there.

With resistance exercises, where the body meets the resistance of weights, bands, or its own weight, we find another vital movement. Here, muscle strength is honed, bone density fortified, and the curtains rise on an enhanced physical performance that transcends the confines of age.

The guidelines advocate dedicating a minimum of 150 minutes weekly to moderate-intensity aerobic exercise or 75 minutes to more vigorous aerobic activity. Additionally, it is advised to incorporate muscle-strengthening exercises for at least two days each week. However, it's crucial to customise the exercise regimen to align with individual capabilities, preferences, and any prevailing health considerations.

Within the realm of well-being, two paramount pillars emerge, the sanctuary of restful sleep and the art of stress mastery. These elements, together, wield a profound influence over our physical and mental health. Proper sleep, parallel to a restorative potion, weaves the threads of optimal functioning and enhanced health. It works its magic, enabling the body to engage in repair and rejuvenation, tissues mend, the immune system fortifies its ramparts, and physical recovery becomes apparent.

Adequate sleep stands as an essential pillar for the nourishment of cognitive faculties, encompassing memory consolidation, learning prowess, unwavering attention, and adept problem-solving abilities. Furthermore, restorative slumber bears a profound influence on emotional fortitude, endowing individuals with heightened resilience in the face of turbulent emotions, the mastery of mood regulation, and a decreased susceptibility to mental health afflictions.

As the inevitable march of time proceeds, the cherished gift of sleep reveals its diverse requisites through life's stages. For those who have ventured into adulthood, the sought-after benchmark lies within the span of 7 to 9 hours of nightly reprieve. In contrast, the burgeoning minds of children and adolescents' hunger for a more generous endowment, seeking in the vicinity of 10 to 12 hours of revitalising respite each day.

Establishing a steadfast sleeping regimen and adhering to a fixed bedtime and wake-up schedule, regulates our body's internal clock. Equally pivotal is the creation of a serene and snug sleeping sanctuary, a chamber draped in darkness, exuding tranquillity, and maintained at an optimal temperature.

In the twilight moments before slumber, a calming prelude is essential. Whether it's the gentle strains of soothing melodies, the pages of a captivating book, the refreshing cascade of a shower, or the serene refuge of meditation, these rituals signal to the body that the hour of rest has arrived.

In our quest for unblemished repose, we must also avoid sleep's adversaries, stimulants like caffeine and nicotine, as well as the siren call of electronic devices that beckon close to bedtime. These intruders, if allowed, may shroud our dreams in unrest, hindering the pursuit of truly restorative sleep.

Stress, a natural reaction to demanding and high-pressure circumstances, serves as an inherent facet of the human experience. Nevertheless, the sustained or excessive presence of stress can cast a shadow upon both our physical and mental well-being, ushering in a waterfall of adverse consequences.

In the quest for equilibrium and enhanced vitality, the mastery of effective stress management techniques emerges as a beacon of hope. Among these methods, a steadfast commitment to a well-rounded diet takes centre stage.

An alimentary regimen that embraces the bounty of whole grains, the vibrance of fruits and vegetables, the sustenance of lean proteins, and the grace of healthy fats becomes a cornerstone of not only nourishing the body but also cultivating resilience in the face of life's inevitable trials. In the sphere of well-being, nutrition stands as an instrument of harmony, soothing the discordant notes of stress and illuminating the path toward a brighter, healthier existence.

In the quest for inner serenity amidst life's chaotic tempest, a repertoire of calming techniques emerges as our guiding lights. These include the gentle pulse of deep breathing exercises, the deliberate release of tension through gradual muscle relaxation, the tranquil embrace of meditation, and the harmonious union of body and spirit in the practice of yoga. Each, in its own way, holds the power to still the turbulent waters of stress, depression, and anxiety, offering solace to the restless mind.

In the intricate tapestry of existence, time weaves a constant thread, often laden with constraints and pressures. To navigate this relentless current, we must cultivate the art of discernment. This entails the skilful act of prioritisation, the wise delegation of responsibilities when necessary, and the artful transformation of complex tasks into smaller, more manageable fragments. In this deliberate act of breaking down the formidable into bite-sized morsels, we untangle the knots of stress woven by time's relentless demands, ushering in a sense of control and mastery over our days.

There exists no fault in seeking solace within the embrace of friends, family, or supportive communities from time to time. These connections offer a sanctuary where concerns find voice and emotional sustenance blossoms. The cultivation of positive and supportive relationships serves as a potent antidote to the looming shadows of stress, depression, or anxiety, casting a warm, protective light upon our emotional landscape.

In our relentless pursuit of life's demands, we often neglect the very essence of our well-being, a grave oversight, indeed. It is incumbent upon us to practise self-care, relaxation, and personal nourishment into the fabric of our existence. To this end, we must ardently engage in hobbies that ignite our spirits, extend the hand of self-compassion to our weary souls, and immerse ourselves in activities that evoke joy and relaxation. This, more than anything else, remains paramount in our quest for a life truly well-lived.

In the tenacious grip of unyielding stress, when it morphs into an unwelcome guest that refuses to depart, intruding upon the sanctity of our daily existence, it is a wise course of action to seek the guidance of seasoned professionals. Among them, healthcare providers and mental health experts stand as sources of optimism, offering a tailored compass to navigate the labyrinthine complexities of individual needs.

In the grand scheme of humanity, we each bear the unique weight of stress, and our responses to its call vary as widely as the colours of a rainbow. The art lies in discovering the strategies that resonate most profoundly with our own souls, for therein lies the key to resilience. Within this intricate mosaic of well-being, slumber takes its rightful place as a cornerstone.

To this end, the pursuit of sound sleep and the deliberate application of stress management techniques compose essential brushstrokes, forming a comprehensive canvas upon which the portrait of enduring physical and mental health is painted.

Pharmaceutical or pharmacological interventions denote the artful deployment of medicinal agents, wielded with the intent to prevent, remedy, or shepherd a diverse array of health conditions. In the insistent pursuit of longevity and vitality, the realm of pharmacological interventions opens a gateway to explore the fine art of sculpting the ageing process into a tapestry of graceful maturation.

Rapamycin, a pharmacological masterpiece that delicately conducts the rhythm of the mechanistic target of the rapamycin (mTOR) pathway. Picture this pathway as a virtuoso, directing the intricate symphony of cell development, metabolism, and the inexorable march of time itself. Yet, with the introduction of rapamycin, this maestro's baton moves with subtle grace, altering the tempo.

The stage, illuminated by a multitude of studies spanning diverse life forms, unveils the spellbinding potential of rapamycin, a potential to elongate the fragile filament of existence and infuse vitality into life's very fabric. In its presence, the haunting spectre of ageing takes on a new direction, its shadow receding to make room for the alluring prospect of a prolonged and healthier journey through the corridors of time.

Metformin, an oral medication renowned for its prowess in enhancing insulin sensitivity and fine-tuning glucose regulation, emerges as a promising elixir in the quest for longevity. Emboldened by the findings of animal studies, Metformin carries the alluring potential to stretch the tapestry of life while curbing the onset of age-related afflictions.

In this pharmaceutical melody, senolytics, a class of drugs designed to seek out and dismantle senescent or ageing cells, takes its rightful place. Their role, akin to a surgeon's precision, offers the tantalising prospect of pruning the branches of cellular decline.

Then, there's Nicotinamide adenine dinucleotide (NAD+), a coenzyme that gracefully choreographs a multitude of cellular processes. Alas, its presence dwindles with the march of time, yet a rekindling of NAD+ levels promise the unfolding of anti-ageing effects. In this pharmacological arena, these remarkable agents, Metformin, senolytics, and NAD+, converge as heralds of a new era. Their collective promise lies in the art of deferring the advent of age-related maladies, holding the keys to robust and healthy ageing.

Chapter 3 - Nurturing a Positive Mindset for Health and Longevity

In the frenetic and at times overwhelming landscape of today's world, the cultivation of a positive mindset stands as a beacon of paramount significance. Its influence ripples through both mental and physical well-being, resonating with profound implications for our health and our lives. Our thoughts and attitudes, it turns out, are architects of our own destiny, wielding the power to shape the contours of our existence.

The embrace of a positive mindset emerges as an invaluable ally, offering the fortitude to navigate life's turbulent waters with grace, alleviating the weight of stress, and bestowing a vibrant quality to our days. The foundation for a life brimming with fulfilment and meaning finds its roots in the nurturing of optimistic thoughts, the daily practice of gratitude, and the diligent engagement in self-care. In this deliberate act of tending to our inner gardens, we sow the seeds of a future blooming with promise and well-being.

A positive mindset isn't merely a state of mind, it is also about optimism, grace under pressure, and the embrace of wholesome habits. It manifests as a mental canvas adorned with the vibrant tones of positivity, resilience, and an unwavering zeal in the face of adversity. Within this mental landscape, the seeds of well-being take root and flourish.

Mental health blooms in its nurturing embrace, while the performance of our daily endeavours soars to new heights. In its gentle glow, life itself takes on a deeper, more fulfilling resonance, painting a portrait of boundless potential and flourishing vitality.

Positive psychology has unveiled a captivating revelation, the influence of an optimistic mindset transcends the boundaries of mere thought, reaching into the very core of our physiology. As the mind dons the robes of positivity, biochemical responses ensue, with neurotransmitters like dopamine and serotonin taking centre stage. These chemical messengers, renowned bearers of cheerfulness and enthusiasm, become emissaries of holistic well-being.

In this transformative mental landscape, the effects ripple far beyond a sunny disposition. Stress, that relentless foe, is subdued, its tempestuous waves stilled. Immune function is invigorated, and the heart beats to the rhythm of improved cardiovascular health. Positive mentality, it seems, conducts a profound concerto of wellness, weaving its harmonious threads through the fabric of our very being.

Positivity transcends mere subjectivity, its impact stretches far and wide across the sphere of well-being, leaving observable imprints in its wake. At its heart lies optimism, a cornerstone of the positive mindset. It is not merely a rosy lens through which life is perceived but a profound commitment to unearthing the gems of positivity even amid life's twists and turns.

Optimistic souls are the unwavering trailblazers in the face of adversity. They stand resolute, fortified by the unwavering belief in their ability to conquer obstacles. To them, hurdles are but fleeting moments in time, not permanent fixtures casting shadows. When we choose the path of optimism, we lay the groundwork for resilience, soothing the tumultuous waves of stress, and opening wide the gates to fresh opportunities.

In this choosing, we set in motion a self-fulfilling prophecy, where our positive beliefs become the architects of our actions and the conductors of the outcomes we encounter. With optimism as our guide, the canvas of life takes on a radiant shade, a testament to the transformative power of positive thinking.

The philosophical connection between a positive mindset and enhanced mental health is an intrinsic bond that holds the key to transformation. In the realm of positivity, we wield the alchemical power to vanquish negative self-talk, to challenge the shackles of limiting beliefs, and to usher in a kinder, more benevolent inner dialogue.

The ripple effect of positive thinking extends far beyond the confines of our thoughts, gently nudging aside the heavy clouds of anxiety and depression, while nurturing the tender sprout of self-worth and emotional well-being. It equips us with the resilient armour of coping strategies, fortifying our ability to gracefully navigate the ever-shifting tides of change and emerge stronger from the depths of setbacks.

In its essence, a positive mindset emerges as the harbinger of a remarkable journey, an unwavering guide that paves the way for success, nurtures personal development, and kindles the fires of great achievement. It is, indeed, a powerful catalyst, beckoning us toward a brighter, more prosperous future.

In the domain of unwavering self-belief and a resolute positive outlook, obstacles transform into steppingstones along the path to accomplishment. When we wholeheartedly embrace our capabilities and talents, when we confront challenges not as burdens but as chances for evolution, our perseverance becomes an unshakable force propelling us toward our goals.

Positive thinkers, by nature, are torchbearers of motivation, artisans of innovation, and experts in resourcefulness. They navigate life's intriguing challenges with an unwavering spirit, unlocking a reservoir of productivity that knows no bounds. Their victories, like radiant stars, illuminate the diverse spheres of existence, from personal relationships to the landscapes of career and education. In their footsteps, we discover the art of not merely surviving but thriving, for positivity begets triumph in the grand symphony of life.

Resilience is the profound capacity to rebound from life's obstacles and adversity, a cornerstone of a buoyant mindset. Optimistic individuals regard setbacks as fleeting hurdles and recognise disappointments as invaluable lessons. They possess the cognitive fortitude to embrace change gracefully and uncover innovative solutions when circumstances demand.

Through the cultivation of resilience, we equip ourselves to navigate the intricate tapestry of life's challenges with greater finesse, preserve our equilibrium, and persevere unwaveringly in the relentless pursuit of our aspirations.

A positive mindset yields benefits not only for individuals but also overwhelmingly shapes their interactions with others. Those who embrace positivity radiate an aura of optimism, drawing kindred spirits into their orbit. The adoption of a positive mindset sets in motion a powerful ripple effect, disseminating confidence and happiness throughout their social spheres. The influence of such a mindset cannot be understated.

Through the nurturing embrace of optimism, we unlock a cascade of transformative effects, enhanced mental well-being, the nurturing of success, the fortification of resilience, and the cultivation of enriching relationships. In doing so, we release our untapped potential and craft a life imbued with profound joy, fulfilment, and purpose.

Every day presents us with an acute choice, one that we can consciously shape and refine. It is the choice to recalibrate our thoughts and feelings, a decision that wields an intricate influence over our physical and emotional well-being. The subtle tendrils of negativity, stress, apprehension, and cynicism, can slyly erode the fortitude of our immune system, elevate the presence of chronic ailments, and impede the innate curative rhythms of our body.

Conversely, the radiance of a positive mindset possesses the transformative capacity to bolster our resilience, nurture the sanctuary of emotional well-being, and, remarkably, accelerate the convalescence journey from ailments or injuries.

The mind-body connection stands as a remarkable phenomenon that has captured significant attention in contemporary times. It underscores the extreme impact our thoughts, emotions, and attitudes wield over our physical health and the journey toward longevity. This intricate spectacle alludes to the complicated interplay between our mental and emotional states, complexly woven into the fabric of our physical well-being.

Cultivating a positive mindset emerges as a potent force in sculpting our holistic well-being, enhancing the defences of our immune system, mitigating the perils of chronic ailments, and nurturing the seeds of a longer, more vibrant life. It is a universally accepted truth that the realm of our thoughts, beliefs, and emotions holds the power to orchestrate complex physiological symphonies, rewriting the production of hormones, the resilience of our immune defences, and the vitality of our cellular operations.

The shadows cast by negative emotions like stress, anxiety, and anger can unfurl a ceaseless banner of chronic inflammation, casting a sombre hue over multiple bodily systems, ultimately paving a path towards heightened vulnerability to afflictions. In stark contrast, the radiance of positive sentiments and an optimistic mindset operates as a catalyst for the release of beneficial hormones, raising a harmonious crescendo within our immune apparatus, and nurturing the fertile grounds of optimal well-being.

The intimate connection between a positive mindset and healthier lifestyle choices is a matter of profound significance. Those who embrace positivity tend to gravitate towards practices that enrich their lives, a commitment to regular exercise, a mindful embrace of a balanced diet, a reverence for restorative sleep, and a steadfast avoidance of detrimental habits like smoking and excessive alcohol consumption.

By consciously nurturing a positive mindset, individuals grant themselves a priceless gift, the gift of enhanced self-worth, and in turn embark on a journey where self-care takes centre stage in their lives.

These virtuous lifestyle practices yield rich benefits bestowing upon us the blessings of improved physical health, diminished vulnerability to chronic maladies, and a lengthened sojourn on the path of longevity. It is a testament to the significant sway our beliefs and expectations wield over the canvas of our health.

Consider the placebo effect, a testament to the alchemical power of belief. It vividly illustrates how the mere conviction in a treatment's efficacy can manifest tangible physiological transformations and symptom amelioration. In similar fashion, individuals who harbour a positive mindset naturally port elevated expectations for their health and recovery, leading to more favourable health outcomes.

By tapping into the reservoir of belief and embracing the radiant energy of positivity, we embark on a voyage that unlocks our innate healing potential, charting a course where our health and longevity become the beneficiaries of our own optimistic influence.

The profound influence of a positive mindset reverberates not only through emotional well-being but also extends its benevolent touch to our physical health. Inhabitants of the sunny realm of optimism often find themselves immersed in the gentle embrace of positive emotions, joy, gratitude, and contentment.

These emotions, akin to celestial orchestrations, are intricately intertwined with improved cardiovascular vigour, the reinforcement of the immune stronghold, and the mitigation of the shadow of chronic afflictions. Through the practice of gratitude, the pursuit of activities that ignite the fires of exhilaration, and the nurturing of meaningful connections, individuals craft the complex tapestry of emotional well-being. They become architects of their own health and stewards of an enduring legacy marked by vitality and longevity.

Having a profound sense of purpose and meaning in one's life stands as a compass guiding us towards improved health and a lengthened journey through the pages of time. Positive thinkers, as if enlightened by a celestial beacon, often find themselves having a clear understanding of their principles and aspirations. This clarity bestows upon them a profound sense of purpose and a steadfast direction.

Through the discernment and pursuit of actions aligned with their passions and values, individuals cultivate a fertile landscape where the seeds of life satisfaction flourish, the burdens of stress dissipate, and the tapestry of overall well-being is artfully woven. In this endeavour, they craft a narrative of vitality and enduring significance.

An essential facet of nurturing a positive mindset resides in the deliberate cultivation of optimism and gratitude. Optimism beckons us to uphold a favourable perspective, channelling our focus toward the rays of positive possibilities. Gratitude, on the other hand, encourages us to unfurl an appreciation for the blessings in our lives, both big and small.

This transformative journey unfolds through actions such as maintaining a gratitude journal to document life's gifts, expressing heartfelt appreciation to those who grace our path, and skilfully recasting adversities into opportunities for profound learning and growth. In these acts, we find the brushstrokes that paint a more vibrant and uplifting mindset.

Engaging in the practices of optimism and gratitude constitutes a revolutionary endeavour, one that holds the potential to intensely enrich our holistic well-being and extend our sojourn through the chapters of life. In the embrace of an optimistic perspective and the warm acknowledgement of gratitude's embrace, we set in motion the gears of positive thought, constructing a solid foundation upon which the tower of an extended, vibrant, and fulfilling life can be erected.

As we welcome the radiance of optimism into our mindset, we fortify the ramparts of our resilience, elevate the contours of our overall well-being, and augment the promise of a lengthened and healthier existence. This journey serves as a testament to the remarkable influence of our thoughts and attitudes on our lives.

The cultivation of a positive mindset is an endeavour that demands deliberate intention and consistent practice. It requires a vigilant awareness of your thoughts and a resolute commitment to steer clear of undesirable or pessimistic thinking patterns. Embrace challenges as steppingstones on the path of personal growth and knowledge acquisition.

Engage in the art of positive self-talk and swap out self-limiting beliefs with empowering affirmations that resonate with your aspirations. Immerse yourself in inspiring literature and seek the company of motivated individuals who fuel your drive for positivity. Over time, these intentional behaviours will construct the scaffolding of a positive mindset, one that not only nurtures well-being but also paves the way toward a longer, more fulfilling life.

Gratitude stands as a potent practice, an alchemy that forges the framework of a positive mindset and exerts a considerable influence upon our well-being. It summons us to perceive, acknowledge, and hold in reverence the myriad blessings that adorn our lives, whether grand or minute.

The habitual cultivation of gratitude acts as a balm, soothing the jagged edges of stress, alleviating the shadows of depression, elevating the sanctuary of emotional well-being, and bestowing the gift of profound life contentment. In the embrace of gratitude, we undergo a transformation of perspective, shifting our gaze from the realm of scarcity to the treasury of abundance that surrounds us. This shift in outlook fosters a penetrating sense of plenitude and satiety, enriching the very fabric of our existence.

Incorporating gratitude into the fabric of our daily existence is paramount for reaping its abundant rewards. To incorporate this virtue into our lives, we must cultivate gratitude as a habitual companion. Commence by embarking on a journey with a gratitude journal, where the painting of thoughts is adorned daily with a few precious moments of appreciation. Deliberately pause to contemplate blessings, either as the sun heralds a new day or as the moon ushers in the night.

Simple expressions of thanks to those who enrich your life serve as beacons of appreciation. Embrace mindfulness, letting it cradle your soul in the gentle embrace of the present moment, where the beauty and goodness of the world reveal themselves. These fundamental practices hold the key to reshaping your perspective, enriching the very essence of your being, and fostering a profound sense of well-being.

The cultivation of optimism and gratitude is a gift that extends far beyond the boundaries of our own lives, touching the hearts of those who orbit around us. Those who bear the mantle of optimism and gratitude become radiant beacons, casting light into the lives of others, lifting their spirits, and igniting the flames of inspiration.

As we nurture this harmonious environment, sowing the seeds of optimism and gratitude into the fertile soil of our interactions, we set in motion a transformative ripple effect that stretches far beyond our own horizons. It becomes a tapestry woven with threads of positivity, painting the world with the colours of hope and appreciation.

The cultivation of positive emotions and meaningful connections unfurls an embroidery of benefits, enriching the bonds within our relationships, bolstering the scaffolding of social support, and elevating the collective well-being of all involved.

To master the art of fostering optimism and gratitude, it is imperative to infuse the spirit of positive thinking into the various facets of our existence. Begin by curating your environment with positive influences, surround yourself with supportive friends, mentors, or role models who embody the virtues of optimism and gratitude.

Engage in activities that kindle joy and a sense of fulfilment, for they are natural catalysts for nurturing positive thoughts. Cherish your physical well-being through a regimen of regular exercise, nourishing foods, and ample rest, recognising that a healthy body forms the bedrock upon which a positive mindset can thrive. In weaving these threads into the fabric of your life, you not only elevate your own existence but also contribute to the flourishing well-being that envelops all who share in your journey.

The profound influence of stress on our overall well-being, encircling both our physical and mental health, cannot be overstated. The cultivation of efficacious stress management techniques assumes paramount importance in generating a buoyant and optimistic mindset.

In this endeavour, an array of methods emerges as potent allies. The art of meditation, with its capacity to bestow tranquillity upon the mind, stands as a formidable bulwark against the ravages of stress. Likewise, the practice of deep breathing exercises offers a soothing relieve to our frazzled nerves, aiding in the restoration of equilibrium.

Physical activity, undertaken with regularity and intent, serves as a stalwart guardian of our health, imbuing us with the resilience to withstand the deleterious effects of stress. Engaging in pursuits that ignite our passions and bring forth joy and fulfilment further contributes to the alchemy of stress management, propelling us towards a more sanguine perspective on life. In sum, the pursuit of stress management, encompassing these time-tested methods, becomes an invaluable cornerstone in the construction of a positive and harmonious existence.

Moreover, the art of nurturing resilience, that remarkable capacity to rebound gracefully in the face of adversity, serves as an invaluable ally in the preservation of a constructive outlook during challenging epochs. In the relentless hustle and unyielding crucible of our modern existence, the adept management of stress and the cultivation of resilience emerge as linchpins, holding the key to our sustained well-being and the pursuit of a long and gratifying life.

The persistent strain of chronic stress exacts a toll on both our physical and mental well-being, while resilience serves as the anchor that allows us to weather adversity and spring back into equilibrium. Through the adept application of stress management strategies and the nurturing of resilience, we enhance our capacity to navigate the trials of existence, reduce the vulnerability to stress-induced ailments, and pave the way for an extended and healthier life.

Prolonged encounters with stress cast a shadow of detriment upon our health and overall well-being. It disrupts the innate equilibrium of our bodies, ushering in heightened inflammation, a compromised immune system, and heightened susceptibility to the chronic afflictions that plague our era, encompassing cardiovascular maladies, diabetes, and the spectre of mental health disorders.

Recognising the profound interplay between stress and longevity underscores the imperative of harnessing effective stress management methodologies. Skilful navigation of stress emerges as an indispensable cornerstone, safeguarding the sanctity of optimal health and fostering the prospect of a protracted and vibrant existence.

Within the arsenal of well-being, an array of techniques and practices stands ready to alleviate the burden of stress. The art of mindfulness, for instance, offers a refuge for the mind, bestowing serenity and temperance upon our tumultuous thoughts, ultimately diminishing the weight of stress.

Likewise, the commitment to regular physical exertion, be it through the gentle pace of walking, the invigorating rhythm of jogging, the expressive artistry of dance, or the contemplative grace of yoga, unleashes a cascade of mood-enhancing molecules, those blissful elixirs of contentment, which serve to dispel the shadows of stress and elevate our spirits.

The art of stress reduction encompasses several facets of proficiency. For instance, setting attainable objectives, mastering time management, and aligning priorities can alleviate the strain wrought by relentless pressure, fostering not only a sense of control but also the sweet taste of success.

Yet, in the sphere of resilience, the importance of social bonds cannot be understated. Establishing a robust support network and nurturing positive relationships weave a safety net of emotional sustenance, inspiration, and a profound sense of belonging, collectively serving as potent shields against the pernicious effects of chronic stress.

Moreover, the domain of relaxation reveals its enchanting therapeutic allure. Methods such as progressive muscle relaxation, the nurturing balm of plant essence therapy, or the humble indulgence in a tranquil bath possess the remarkable ability to rouse the body's inborn response to relaxation. They gently unfurl its soothing wings, ushering away the tempestuous clouds of stress with a tender grace.

Cultivating a positive mindset requires a deliberate shift in perspective, one that transforms challenges into steppingstones for personal growth, redirects attention towards solutions rather than dwelling on problems, and constructs a foundation of optimism.

By giving precedence to self-renewal practices, such as immersing oneself in leisurely pursuits, mastering the art of relaxation, ensuring an ample supply of restorative sleep, and embracing a wholesome lifestyle, we replenish our inner reservoirs of vitality. This, in turn, fortifies our resilience and contributes to a flourishing state of overall well-being.

Turning to the embrace of family, friends, or qualified professionals in times of adversity not only fosters resilience but also bestows upon us an invaluable wellspring of additional resources to navigate the trials we encounter. In parallel, honing the art of critical problem-solving equips us to confront challenges with a proactive stance, disassembling them into digestible components and uncovering tangible solutions along the way.

Our surroundings, both the physical and social landscapes we inhabit, wield profound influence over our mindset. Thus, the company we keep should consist of individuals radiating cheerfulness, offering unwavering support, and serving as wellsprings of motivation and inspiration.

Equally vital is the creation of a nurturing physical environment, one meticulously tailored to integrate elements that exude happiness and serenity through streamlined organisation. The act of sculpting such a positive and supportive environment assumes a role of immense significance, for it becomes a catalyst for the cultivation of longevity and holistic well-being. The presence of positivity in our surroundings acts as a potent tonic, reducing the weight of stress, fortifying our resilience, and nurturing the fertile soil from which a healthier mindset may flourish.

Our physical and mental well-being are intricately connected to the fabric of our social bonds, surroundings, and daily encounters. Environments steeped in negativity, with their burdens of stress, toxicity, and pessimism, become fertile grounds for elevated stress levels, compromised mental health, and the onset of chronic ailments. In stark contrast, positive environments, where enthusiasm, support, and wholesome pursuits thrive, emerge as potent antidotes.

They not only bolster our resilience but also alleviate the weight of stress, thereby nurturing the promise of an extended and healthier existence. At the heart of forging such a nurturing environment lies the cornerstone of positive relationships, a fundamental force that shapes the landscape of care and support.

Detrimental influences possess the power to obstruct both well-being and the pursuit of a prolonged life. To safeguard one's vitality, it becomes imperative to enact a deliberate separation from relationships, circumstances, or settings that perpetually usher in negativity, strain, or harm. This entails the establishment of firm boundaries with those who exude negativity, a judicious limitation of exposure to adverse influences, and a conscientious awareness of the profound impact certain environments can wield upon our mental and emotional equilibrium.

As we diminish our contact with detrimental forces, we liberate precious space for the blossoming of positivity. Moreover, the physical landscapes that envelop us wield a palpable sway over our mood and overall well-being. Therefore, it becomes an essential endeavour to craft a physical environment that radiates positivity, one that acts as a steadfast ally in our quest for longevity and lasting contentment.

The allure of an uncluttered space lies in its ability to bestow serenity and foster clarity. By decluttering and meticulously organising your living and working spaces, you orchestrate an atmosphere of tranquil efficiency that sharpens focus and alleviates the weight of stress.

Moreover, the tender embrace of nature beckons as an oasis of solace. It is advisable to immerse oneself in the great outdoors whenever possible, letting the open air breathe life into one's spirit. Additionally, infusing your environment with natural elements, those harbingers of relaxation and well-being, can work wonders for the mind and soul.

Embrace the practice of adorning your surroundings with items and decorations that radiate peace, joy, and motivation. Let the walls of your space tell stories of inspiration through the display of cherished photographs, uplifting artwork, or daily affirmations that elevate your spirits and evoke memories of positive experiences.

Craft an ambiance of serenity by employing soothing colours, tuning into tranquil melodies, and introducing the soothing touch of aromatherapy. The art of infusing your daily life with these elements of positivity wields remarkable influence over your health, well-being, and the potential for a longer and more fulfilling life.

In the relentless pursuit of health and a long life, our attention typically gravitates towards external factors such as diet, exercise, and medical care. Yet, there exists a pivotal element that often eludes the spotlight, the art of self-compassion. Self-compassion is, at its core, the gentle act of being kind to ourselves.

It entails the cultivation of a nurturing and supportive relationship with our own selves, serving as a vessel in which resilience is forged and the foundations of overall well-being are laid. In this often-overlooked practice lies a profound wellspring of health and longevity.

This practice comprises three fundamental pillars, self-kindness, common humanity, and mindfulness. It commences with the gentle act of extending understanding and compassion to ourselves, shunning self-criticism and self-condemnation. At its core, it involves treating ourselves with the same tenderness and support we would readily offer to a beloved friend in their time of need.

Embracing the reality that suffering and adversity are intrinsic to the human experience paves the path to nurturing self-compassion. Acknowledging that our struggles are not solitary, that failures are a shared human experience, fosters a profound sense of connection and empathy. At the heart of this practice lies mindfulness, a state of being fully present and attuned to our thoughts, emotions, and physical sensations, all without the burden of judgment.

Self-compassion empowers us to bear witness to our experiences with a profound empathy, and in doing so, it enables responses that are devoid of reactivity and judgment. This nurturing embrace of self-kindness serves as a defence for our stress-laden souls, offering a sympathetic and understanding reaction to our own trials. As a result, we navigate challenging times with increased grace and resilience, cultivating a landscape of emotional well-being where self-acceptance, self-worth, and self-love flourish.

Within this gentle cocoon of self-compassion, we forge positive coping strategies that bolster our emotional resilience. It becomes a steadfast companion on the journey to physical health, encouraging the adoption of salubrious lifestyle choices while diminishing the allure of unhealthy coping mechanisms.

In its radiant presence, a more positive attitude towards self-care blooms, illuminating the path to a life imbued with vitality and well-being. When we extend kindness and empathy to ourselves, we lay the foundation for fostering positive and fulfilling relationships with others. To truly nurture self-compassion in one's life, it becomes imperative to clothe oneself in a gentle, kind-hearted disposition, especially during those moments of inner turmoil or self-critique.

Replace the habit of self-critique with a steady flow of self-encouragement and self-love. Elevate self-care to a sacred ritual that nourishes your physical, mental, and emotional well-being. Engage in activities that evoke joy, relaxation, and rejuvenation. Make mindfulness a constant companion, nurturing your ability to observe thoughts and emotions without harsh judgment. Approach life's experiences with curiosity, enthusiasm, and a heart filled with compassion.

Forge a daily practice of positive self-talk, substituting self-critical thoughts with gentle and empathetic affirmations. Speak words of wisdom and encouragement to yourself, always be mindful of your inherent worth. Acknowledge that facing adversity and setbacks is part of the human journey and respond with self-compassion and self-acceptance. In moments of need, do not hesitate to seek support or guidance from loved ones or professionals. Surround yourself with individuals who uplift and empower you, creating a circle of positivity that nurtures your well-being and fuels your journey towards self-compassion.

Chapter 4 - The Power of Nutritious Eating: Fuelling Your Body for Life

Amidst the frenetic pace of contemporary life, replete with an array of convenient fast-food choices and relentlessly stressful environments, the inclination to neglect our bodies is a pervasive temptation. Yet, we must not underestimate the pivotal role played by the sustenance we partake in each day. This nourishment serves as the essential fuel that propels our exquisitely designed bodies toward health and well-being.

The significance of our dietary choices extends beyond the mere act of consuming the right foods. It entails a profound transformation in our relationship with sustenance, a redefinition of what it means to experience true nourishment. Equipping ourselves with knowledge and crafting strategies that enable informed food decisions becomes paramount, as these choices hold the potential to decisively influence our health and longevity.

The potency of nutritious eating is undeniable, for it possesses the remarkable ability not only to restore and energise but also to chart new trajectories for our lives. In this journey toward nourishment, we unearth a wellspring of transformative power that has the capacity to reshape our very existence.

Food stands as a requisite element for the sustenance and optimal operation of our bodies. It serves as the fundamental source of energy and vital nutrients necessary for the intricate processes of growth, repair, and the maintenance of bodily functions. To navigate the terrain of nutrition is to gain insight into the mechanisms that govern our relationship with food, thereby empowering us to make enlightened dietary choices that have the potential to foster health and overall well-being.

Carbohydrates reign supreme as the body's primary source of energy, and they encompass sugars, starches, and dietary fibres within their ranks. Simple carbohydrates, such as sugars, grace us with their presence in fruits, milk, and processed foods. In contrast, complex carbohydrates, typified by starches, make their home in grains, beans, and an assortment of vegetables.

The role of carbohydrates extends far beyond mere energy provision. They play a pivotal part in the regulation of blood glucose levels. Moreover, they are indispensable for the optimal functioning of the brain, performance during physical activities, and the successful execution of our everyday pursuits.

Proteins serve as the cornerstone for constructing and mending tissues, as well as crafting essential molecules, enzymes, and hormones within our bodies. Within the realm of proteins, we encounter a palette of twenty distinct amino acids, each assuming the role of a foundational building block.

Among these twenty amino acids, our bodies wield the remarkable ability to independently synthesise eleven. These self-made amino acids are aptly termed non-essential, for our systems possess the intrinsic capability to produce them internally, thereby rendering them indispensable but not reliant on external sources.

Nonetheless, within the realm of amino acids, there exist nine indispensable players, ones our bodies are incapable of producing autonomously. These vital components are known as essential amino acids. To secure a complete arsenal of these essential building blocks for proper growth, repair, and functioning, it becomes imperative to diversify our protein intake.

The blueprint for a well-rounded diet hinge on the inclusion of a wide spectrum of protein sources. This dietary tapestry, adorned with foods such as meat, fish, dairy products, legumes, nuts, and seeds, ensures that our bodies receive the full complement of essential amino acids they require to thrive.

Proteins stand as stalwart defenders of immune function, essential players in the preservation of muscle mass, and key actors in a myriad of biochemical processes. On the other front, fats emerge as another formidable source of energy, executing critical roles in nutrient absorption, hormone synthesis, and the structure of cell membranes.

Within the dominion of fats, we encounter a trio of distinct characters, saturated fats, predominantly nestled within animal products, unsaturated fats, which find their home in plant oils, nuts, and seeds and the notorious trans fats, often lurking within the folds of processed foods.

The sage counsel dictates a diet that tilts toward the consumption of wholesome unsaturated fats, while maintaining a vigilant watch against the infiltration of trans fats and excessive saturated fats. Embracing the bounty of healthy fats, we usher in a symphony of benefits for our cardiovascular health, lend a hand in regulating body temperature, and offer sustenance to the intricate machinery of brain function.

Vitamins, the organic compounds that coordinate a multitude of biochemical processes within the body, assume the role of indispensable coenzymes, facilitating crucial chemical reactions. They are categorised into two groups, water-soluble vitamins, which include vitamin C and the various B vitamins, and fat-soluble vitamins, encompassing vitamins A, D, E, and K.

Each vitamin carries a unique portfolio of responsibilities and can be found in a wide array of foods. These micronutrients champion diverse functions within the body, from bolstering the immune system and nurturing healthy skin to playing pivotal roles in energy metabolism, vision, bone health, and blood clotting.

Minerals, those inorganic elements bestowed by nature, stand as the unheralded architects of crucial bodily functions, including the fortification of bones, the orchestration of nerve activities, and the delicate equilibrium of fluid levels. This illustrious group includes luminaries like selenium, iron, zinc, calcium, potassium, and magnesium, each with its unique sphere of influence. As we partake in various foods, we unknowingly access distinct mineral troves.

These invaluable micronutrients, essential for a gamut of functions encompassing bone health, nerve signalling, muscle contractions, oxygen transport, and the catalytic magic of enzymes, compose an elemental masterpiece that underpins our well-being.

Water, though frequently relegated to the shadows, holds an invaluable role within our dietary mosaic. It choreographs a symphony of physiological processes, deftly orchestrating temperature regulation, aiding in digestion, facilitating the transport of nutrients, and expediting the disposal of waste. Maintaining adequate hydration emerges as a hub for the collage of health and well-being that envelops our lives.

Dietary fibre, a unique form of carbohydrate that eludes full digestion by our bodies, emerges as a basis of digestive well-being. Its role is twofold, it champions the cause of normal bowel movements, ensuring the avoidance of constipation. Fibre is rich and diverse, residing in seeds, fruits, whole grains, vegetables, and nuts.

Antioxidants, on the other hand, stand as vigilant sentinels guarding our body's cells against the ravages wrought by free radicals. These protective compounds are scattered throughout a variety of foods, with vibrant and colourful fruits and vegetables serving as veritable treasure troves of these health-preserving elements.

Food processing encompasses the intricate array of techniques deployed to transform raw ingredients into delectable, consumable food products. With this culinary approach, the very essence of taste, texture, and shelf life is often enhanced. However, certain processing methods wield the power to diminish the nutritional value of food. In their quest for refinement, they may inadvertently strip away dietary fibre or select vitamins, subtly altering the food's nutritional composition.

A well-rounded diet weaves together a medley of foods hailing from a spectrum of diverse food groups. This intricate culinary tapestry is carefully crafted to guarantee the ample intake of all essential nutrients, a vital cornerstone of good health.

Within this mosaic of nutrition, the inclusion of a diverse array of fruits, whole grains, vegetables, wholesome fats, and lean proteins becomes paramount. Knowledge and understanding of the components of food serves as a compass, guiding us toward enlightened dietary decisions that are grounded in knowledge and nourishing to our bodies.

Nutrients stand as the vital building blocks, imperative for the sustenance of good health and the seamless functioning of our bodies. These essential compounds fall into two overarching categories, macronutrients, and micronutrients, each contributing distinct roles to an intricate web of physiological processes.

Macronutrients, the formidable trio that our bodies require in substantial quantities, serve as the fuel and framework for a multitude of bodily functions. These primary players encompass carbohydrates, proteins, and fats, each extending their indispensable contributions to the intricacies of our well-being.

Micronutrients, those essential nutrients sought in smaller quantities when compared to their macronutrient counterparts, bear equal significance in the grand sphere of proper growth, development, and holistic well-being. Nestled within this category are the heralded champions, vitamins, and minerals, each adorned with a multifaceted crown of pivotal roles in an intricate ballet of physiological processes. Together, macronutrients and micronutrients stand as the foundation of our bodily harmony, ensuring the seamless coordination of functions that underpin our existence.

Nutrition assumes a critical role in fortifying the immune system, enhancing its prowess in combatting infections, and upholding holistic well-being. At the heart of this complex mechanism lies the essential role of proteins. These remarkable molecules serve as the architects behind the creation of antibodies, those remarkable sentinels that guide the immune system in its mission to recognise and disarm invasive threats.

By maintaining an ample supply of proteins, we furnish our bodies with the fundamental elements required to scheme a robust immune response, safeguarding our health with unwavering vigilance.

Carbohydrates serve as the vital fuel that empowers our immune cells to carry out their duties with precision and effectiveness. In this symphony of nourishment, it is the whole grains and complex carbohydrates that shine as the champions of sustaining energy levels and fortifying the immune system.

Vitamin C, a formidable ally in the realm of antioxidants steps forward to bolster numerous immune functions, coordinating a harmonious defence. Among its many virtuous deeds, it acts as a catalyst, enhancing the production of white blood cells, the stalwart guardians that stand resolute against the onslaught of infections.

In this rich embroidery of nutrition, we find our sources of Vitamin C in the vibrant varieties of citrus fruits, the succulence of berries, the exotic allure of kiwi, and the crisp vibrancy of bell peppers. They are the instruments of health, playing their part in our body's enduring quest for vitality and well-being.

Vitamin D assumes a pivotal role in the coordination of our immune system, fine-tuning its performance and ensuring the harmonious function of immune cells. It's a guardian against the perils of respiratory infections, with ample vitamin D levels serving as a shield, reducing the risk of such maladies. Nature's spotlight falls on both sunlight and nourishment from the culinary orbit, particularly in the form of fatty fish and dairy products, as sources that bestow this essential nutrient upon us.

Vitamin A, a virtuoso in the realm of health, takes the stage to fortify our skin's defences and bolster the protective ramparts of our mucosal barriers, the sentinel guardians at the body's gates. This nutrient's ability does not end there, it extends to the nurturing and fine-tuning of our immune cells, guiding them to their zenith of performance. This culinary palette unfolds with a vibrant spectrum of offerings, featuring the likes of carrots, sweet potatoes, the verdant embrace of spinach, and the liver's nourishing bounty, all rich reservoirs of this vital nutrient.

In the intricacies of immune function, zinc emerges as a crucial conductor, orchestrating the harmonious interplay of immune cells and ensuring the precision of the immune response. This vital mineral finds its place of honour in nourishing edibles like oysters, beef, nuts, and seeds.

Selenium, a trace mineral endowed with the mantle of an antioxidant guardian, its role is to stand guard, safeguarding the integrity of immune cell function. It takes its place in the pantry of nature, nestled among the treasures of Brazil nuts, the bounty of the deep in fish, and the enduring sustenance of whole grains.

As our immune forces engage in the ceaseless battle against invaders, they are not left defenceless. The armoury of antioxidants, including the likes of vitamins C and E, the golden essence of beta-carotene, and the steadfast selenium, forms an unyielding shield against the onslaught of free radicals.

These guardians of well-being are generously bequeathed upon us by nature's bounty, found in the vibrant array of fruits, verdant vegetables, and the nourishing troves of nuts and seeds.

In their presence, our immune fortifications stand strong, ever ready to face the challenges of the world.

In the intricate complexities of immune vitality, one must not overlook the critical role of proper hydration. Water, the life-giving elixir, serves as a diligent courier, ferrying essential nutrients to our sentry immune cells while assisting in the elegant expulsion of waste from our corporeal abode.

Yet, in this delicate balance, we find that certain dietary culprits conspire against our immune guardians. Excessive sugar, the siren calls of unhealthy fats, and the allure of alcohol can, alas, shroud the immune system in lethargy. The path to resilience lies in judicious restraint, a temperance that confers upon us the gift of a fortified immune stronghold.

In the delicate art of nourishment, portion size emerges as the brushstroke that paints the image of our dietary choices. It wields noteworthy influence over the harmony of our sustenance and the instrumentation of our well-being. With precision akin to a maestro's wand, portion control guides us to partake in a sonata of nutrition, ensuring that we imbibe the essential nutrients in measured doses, free from the cacophony of overindulgence.

In this culinary ballet, the spotlight falls upon caloric equilibrium. To dance in step with our body's needs is to maintain the balance of caloric intake, a tango between sustenance and expenditure. An excess of calories, uninvited and unchecked, may lead to an unwelcome guest, the weight of excess, while a dearth of calories leaves us lighter, perhaps, but devoid of essential nourishment. In the careful choreography of portion size, we find the key to this intricate balance, harmonising our intake with the rhythms of our body's demands.

In the culinary realm, the art of portion control is critical, it orchestrates a delicate balance of macronutrients (carbohydrates, proteins, fats) and the intricate notes of micronutrients (vitamins and minerals). It ensures that the body's grand performance is fuelled with precision.

Consider, for a moment, the digestive system, a stage for the intricate jazz of sustenance. Imposing oversized portions upon this delicate theatre may lead to a dissonance of discomfort and indigestion, a discord in the gastronomic opera. In contrast, the genius of portion mastery results in efficient digestion, allowing each nutrient to shine in its spotlight.

Yet, the significance of this culinary ace extends beyond mere gastronomic finesse. For those navigating the labyrinth of diabetes or insulin resistance, portion control assumes even greater import. It wields the power to harmonise blood sugar levels, a strategy of health that dances to the beat of moderation. Portion control emerges as a frontrunner, ensuring that the body's metabolic opus plays on with grace and balance.

In the jurisdiction of mindful dining, the first stanza is written on the print of food labels, where serving sizes tell the secrets of appropriate portions. It is a code that guides us through the gastronomic maze. Yet, the art of portion control extends beyond labels and numbers. In the culinary arena, smaller portions tell tales of mastery. By choosing diminutive dishes, we create a visual that curbs overindulgence, transforming every bite into a sonnet of satisfaction.

Listen to the hints of your body, for it knows when the final note has been played. The crescendo of contentment is the cue to set down the fork, not when the body groans under the weight of excess. And when the restaurant's offerings resemble an epic saga, remember the power of camaraderie. Sharing is the transformation that transmutes a mound into a manageable feast or a culinary voyage into a shared odyssey.

Cultivate the art of mindful dining, savouring each morsel with deliberate intent and embracing the unhurried pace. In this graceful cadence, your brain finds its voice, signalling the moment of fullness, preventing overindulgence. Embark on a culinary journey that traverses the diverse landscapes of food groups, where variety becomes your compass. This gastronomic expedition brings forth a cornucopia of health rewards, ensuring that your body receives a rich embroidery of essential nutrients.

Within the domain of nutrition, it's a balanced masterpiece of diversity that we seek. Each food, a unique instrument, contributes its own melodic blend of nutrients, vitamins, minerals, antioxidants, and vital compounds, to the grand composition of well-being.

In winding this elaborate collage of flavours, we safeguard ourselves against the ghosts of nutrient deficiencies, for in variety, we find our protection. This assortment of sustenance paints a balanced diet, where the notes of proteins, fats, carbohydrates, and the spectrum of vitamins and minerals unite in perfect harmony.

In the grand composition of wellness, this equilibrium stands as the composer, directing optimal bodily performance and the concerto of overall well-being. A tessellation of diversity in your diet not only wards off the drudgery of culinary routine but also transforms meals into a delight of the senses. Venture into uncharted culinary territories, where new foods and recipes unfold as chapters of excitement in your gastronomic journey.

Each bite becomes a poetic commentary, each dish a thrilling experience, composing a vibrant ode to your dining experience. And beneath this culinary kaleidoscope lies the secret garden of your intestinal flora, where diverse nourishment cultivates a flourishing community of beneficial gut bacteria. In this thriving microcosm, the harmony of well-being finds its echo, resonating with health and vitality.

In the sophisticated landscape of our gut, harmonious and balanced microbes choreograph a masterpiece of functions. Together, they harmonise digestion, reinforce our immunity, and even contribute to the delicate play of our emotions. This instrumentation holds particular significance for those navigating the tangle of food allergies or sensitivities.

The palette of our nutrition expands when we embrace a diverse array of foods. Within this rich drapery, we find the nourishment needed to sustain the body, fulfilling its nutritional prerequisites, where the gut thrives, and the body flourishes.

In the area of nutrition, a diverse culinary approach emerges as a potent shield against the enduring threats of chronic afflictions, such as cardiovascular ailments, diabetes, and specific varieties of cancer. It stands as the guard of balance, preserving a coveted body weight and safeguarding against nutrient deficiencies.

Yet, within this mosaic of nourishment, certain key nutrients like the virtuous omega-3 fatty acids, the invaluable B-vitamins, the steadfast zinc, the fortifying iron, and the tranquilising magnesium, have come under the spotlight. They are not just guardians of physical health but also champions in the dominion of mental well-being, fashioning a tapestry of vitality that extends beyond the body to nurture the very essence of our minds.

Insufficient quantities of these essential nutrients have been correlated with heightened vulnerability to mental health conditions, including depression, anxiety, and cognitive decline. The intricate interplay between the gut and the brain, known as the gut-brain axis, stands as a pivotal factor in mental well-being.

At the heart of this intricate connection lies the gut microbiota, an expansive community of microorganisms that reside within the digestive system and play a paramount role. A diet abundant in fibre and a diverse array of plant-based foods cultivates a flourishing gut microbiome, thereby harmonising with more favourable mental health prospects.

Omega-3 fatty acids, particularly EPA (eicosapentaenoic acid) and DHA (docosahexaenoic acid), assume a significant role in the preservation of cognitive well-being. Their indispensability lies in their capacity to facilitate communication among nerve cells and mitigate inflammation. The inclusion of foods such as fatty fish, walnuts, and flaxseeds in one's diet may yield beneficial impacts on mood and overall mental wellness.

The Mediterranean diet, characterised by its emphasis on the consumption of vegetables, fruits, olive oil, seeds, whole grains, nuts, and moderate portions of dairy, fish, and poultry, has been linked to enhanced mental well-being. This dietary pattern provides a wealth of essential nutrients and fosters a thriving gut microbiome. Within this culinary framework, antioxidants, abundantly present in fruits and vegetables, serve as guardians of the brain, shielding it from oxidative harm and potentially mitigating cognitive decline.

Persistent bodily inflammation has been associated with the emergence of mental health conditions. A diet abundant in processed edibles, sugary substances, and unfavourable fats has the potential to trigger inflammation. In contrast, an anti-inflammatory dietary approach abundant in fruits, veggies, whole grains, and nourishing fats may contribute to the mitigation of inflammation and the enhancement of emotional welfare.

Overindulgence in sugar and intensively processed nourishment has been correlated with heightened susceptibility to depression and anxiety. These consumables can induce abrupt fluctuations in blood sugar, influencing mood and energy levels. The link between diet and mental health is complicated.

In preserving one's mental equilibrium, the significance of a well-rounded diet cannot be overemphasised. A dietary regimen characterised by the inclusion of whole grains, an assortment of fruits, lean proteins, an abundance of vegetables, and the enfold of healthful fats, alongside the indispensable practice of staying adequately hydrated, stands as a paramount endeavour.

It becomes increasingly evident that lapses in nutrition, the persistent scourge of chronic inflammation, and an imbalanced dietary course are intrinsically linked to an elevated vulnerability to mental health afflictions. Therefore, fostering a dietary landscape enriched with essential nutrients and fostering a harmonious ecosystem of gut bacteria may yield significant benefits in the realm of cognitive function, mood modulation, and the holistic panorama of mental well-being.

It is of utmost import to recognise the essential role that diet plays in the sphere of mental health care. This recognition, this acknowledgment, is a non-negotiable foundation in the edifice of mental well-being.

In the area of dietary choices, a multitude of regimens exists, each vying to enhance well-being, control weight, or attain precise fitness aspirations. Every dietary path is endowed with its distinct set of guiding principles, inherent constraints, and proclaimed advantages. Among the array of prominent choices stand the Ketogenic diet, Intermittent Fasting, and the philosophy of Veganism.

The Ketogenic diet, characterised by its high-fat and low-carbohydrate composition, seeks to orchestrate a fundamental shift in the body's primary energy source. This metabolic transformation, known as ketosis, entails the production of ketones, which serve as an alternative fuel reservoir for the body.

In pursuit of this biochemical alteration, the Ketogenic diet imposes constraints on the consumption of high-carbohydrate fare, relegating items such as fruits, grains, select vegetables, legumes, and sugary confections to the dietary side lines. Instead, it accentuates the incorporation of foods such as fish, meat, oils, eggs, seeds, nuts, and low-carbohydrate vegetables into its culinary setting.

Proponents of the ketogenic lifestyle contend that this dietary approach holds the potential to not only facilitate weight loss but also to ameliorate blood sugar control, elevate energy reserves, and bolster mental well-being. Moreover, there is a school of thought that posits the ketogenic diet as a valuable intervention for certain neurological ailments.

However, it's essential to acknowledge that embarking on the keto journey may entail an initial adjustment period marked by transient side effects often dubbed the "keto flu," as the body undergoes the modification to a fat-burning metabolism. It's imperative to recognise that the ketogenic regimen, while promising, may not be universally suitable. The stringent constraints it imposes and the potential for nutritional imbalances may render it challenging for some individuals to sustain over the long term.

Intermittent Fasting, a dietary practice, involves the alternating sequence of nourishment and abstention from food consumption. It's akin to granting the body a respite from its regular dietary routine. While there exist several approaches to this dietary regimen, two of the more prevalent methods include the 16/8 and 5:2 protocols. Under the 16/8 regimen, one abstains from food for a duration of 16 hours, followed by an allotted 8-hour window for eating.

The 5:2 method, on the other hand, adheres to a schedule in which you maintain your regular eating habits for five days of the week, while deliberately curtailing your calorie intake on the remaining two consecutive days. In this approach, fasting, in the traditional sense, isn't the primary objective, instead, the emphasis lies in a reduction of overall caloric consumption.

During these calorie-restricted periods, hydration is encouraged, permitting the consumption of water, tea, or coffee. Though, it's crucial to note that these beverages should be enjoyed without the addition of sugar or milk, ensuring a minimal caloric intake is maintained.

In this dietary methodology, the focus predominantly revolves around the timing of meals, as there are no imposed constraints or restrictions on the variety of foods one may consume. Nevertheless, it remains paramount to underscore the significance of adhering to a balanced and healthful diet. Advocates of intermittent fasting assert a myriad of potential benefits, including assistance in weight management, the enhancement of metabolic functions, support for mental well-being, and a tantalising prospect of potentially extending one's lifespan.

Intermittent fasting emerges as a formidable tool in the quest to regulate blood sugar levels, nurture cardiovascular well-being, and optimise the intricate cellular mechanisms at play within the body. However, it is essential to emphasise that intermittent fasting may not be universally advantageous. This approach is not advised for individuals grappling with chronic health conditions, those who have previously encountered difficulties with their eating patterns, as well as pregnant or breastfeeding women, for whom alternative dietary strategies may be more suitable.

A vegan diet is inherently plant-centric, advocating the complete exclusion of all animal-derived fare, including dairy, eggs, meat, and even honey. In its resolute commitment to plant-based sustenance, this dietary philosophy centres on the consumption of vegetables, fruits, grains, legumes, nuts, seeds, and innovative plant-based substitutes designed to mimic traditional animal products.

The tenets of veganism rigidly eschew any trace of animal products or their derivatives. Remarkably, adherents of this lifestyle often enjoy the added benefit of a diminished susceptibility to chronic ailments such as heart disease, hypertension, and type 2 diabetes mellitus, attesting to the profound impact of their dietary choices on long-term health.

Every dietary regimen carries with it its own set of principles, limitations, and potential advantages. While many individuals may indeed experience success and enhanced well-being through these diets, it remains imperative to approach them with thoughtful deliberation and a commitment to personalisation. The uniqueness of each person's nutritional needs, influenced by factors such as age, activity level, gender, and existing health conditions, highlights the importance of a tailored approach.

Before embarking on any dietary journey, it is of paramount importance to seek guidance from a qualified healthcare professional or registered dietitian. Their expertise can be instrumental in determining the most suitable and effective approach to align with one's health objectives and overall state of well-being. It is crucial to remember that at the foundation of good health lies a balanced and diversified diet, one that provides all the requisite nutrients necessary for overall well-being.

Blue Zones are enclaves across the globe renowned for fostering remarkably long and vibrant lives. These regions, such as Okinawa in Japan, Sardinia in Italy, Nicoya in Costa Rica, Ikaria in Greece, and Loma Linda in California, USA, have gained international acclaim for their inhabitants' exceptional longevity and robust health. The lifestyles and dietary choices of these communities have become subjects of fascination and admiration, owing to their profound association with longevity and overall well-being.

Central to the Blue Zone ethos is a dietary pattern that places paramount importance on the consumption of an abundant array of vegetables. This includes leafy greens, cruciferous vegetables, and a vibrant spectrum of produce rich in colour and vitality. These vegetables serve as veritable powerhouses, teeming with essential vitamins, minerals, and antioxidants that serve as pillars of holistic health.

Additionally, legumes, edible seeds, and the venerable Bengal gram or gram beans constitute dietary cornerstones in many Blue Zone territories. These humble yet nutrient-dense ingredients stand as exemplary sources of plant-based proteins, dietary fibre, and a profusion of vital nutrients, further reinforcing the nutritional wisdom that underpins the Blue Zone way of life.

In the communities inhabiting Blue Zone regions, whole grains occupy a significant place on the plate. Staples like brown rice, quinoa, barley, and oats are cherished for their capacity to bestow enduring vitality and essential nutrients upon those who partake in them. In Mediterranean Blue Zones, like Sardinia and Ikaria, the keystone of their dietary wisdom is none other than the revered olive oil.

Renowned for its abundance of heart-healthy monounsaturated fats and a wealth of antioxidants, olive oil emerges as the principal source of healthy fats in these societies, where it plays a pivotal role in nurturing both well-being and longevity.

Within Blue Zone communities, a familiar presence on their menus comes in the form of nuts and seeds, including sesame seeds, almonds, and walnuts. These modest yet nutritionally potent offerings deliver a trifecta of benefits, healthy fats, protein, and a diverse array of vital nutrients. In coastal Blue Zones such as Okinawa and Sardinia, a measured inclusion of fish and seafood enriches their diets. These oceanic treasures serve as exceptional sources of omega-3 fatty acids, renowned for their role in nurturing heart health and bolstering cognitive function.

In the heart of Blue Zone communities, herbal teas and brews reign supreme as the beverages of choice. Notable instances include the prevalence of green tea in Okinawa and the cherished tradition of savouring wild herb teas in Ikaria. These liquid elixirs bestow upon their drinkers a generous bounty of antioxidants and an assortment of other vital compounds, enriching the body's well-being.

Furthermore, in the Blue Zones of Sardinia and Ikaria, a time-honoured custom of judicious alcohol consumption, particularly in the form of red wine, finds favour. When enjoyed in moderation, red wine unveils its potential cardiovascular benefits, adding a touch of healthful indulgence to these communities' distinctive way of life.

The act of communal dining emerges as a cherished tradition in blue zone areas. Regularly sharing meals with friends and family not only nourishes the body but also nurtures an acute sense of belonging and wellness within the group. In these close-knit societies, mindful eating prevails as a practiced art, allowing individuals to relish their meals without the burden of excessive fullness.

Caloric equilibrium takes centre stage, this emphasis on balanced intake serves as a safeguard against overindulgence and the maintenance of a healthy weight. By incorporating elements of these dietary practices from Blue Zone regions into our own lives, alongside an active and harmonious lifestyle, we may find ourselves on a path towards enhanced overall health and well-being.

The gastrointestinal (GI) tract, colloquially known as the gut, comprises a sophisticated physiological system which is tasked with the breakdown and absorption of nutrients obtained from ingested sustenance. Beyond its fundamental digestive role, incipient investigations underscore the pivotal role of gut health in the broader sphere of holistic well-being, wielding a substantial influence on diverse facets of human physiology encompassing immunological prowess, emotional equilibrium, and the modulation of inflammatory responses.

The gut accommodates a myriad of microorganisms in the order of trillions, collectively designated as the gut microbiome. This sophisticated consortia of bacteria, fungi, viruses, and assorted microorganisms assumes an indispensable mantle in the maintenance of gut homeostasis and by extension, general physiological equilibrium.

The diversely composed and harmonised gut microbiome evinces a correlative association with optimised processes of digestion, assimilation of nutrients, immune competency, and fortification against pathogenic incursions.

An optimally functioning gastrointestinal tract ensures the efficient breakdown and absorption of nutrients derived from ingested food, thereby facilitating the intake of essential vitamins, minerals, and other imperative nutrients vital for sustaining optimal physiological processes.

Within the confines of the gastrointestinal environment, a sizeable portion of the immune system takes residence. The presence of a harmoniously balanced gut microbiome contributes to a meticulously orchestrated immune response, thereby bolstering the body's resilience against the onslaught of infections and maladies.

Furthermore, the intricate interplay between the gut and the central nervous system is orchestrated via the conduit of the gut-brain axis. Notably, the cultivation of a thriving gut microbiome correlates with an elevated state of mental well-being, potentially mitigating the susceptibility to conditions such as anxiety and depression.

Additionally, the presence of a well-balanced gut microbiome imparts a regulatory influence on systemic inflammation. Given that prolonged inflammatory states are intricately linked to an array of chronic ailments, the sustenance of a healthy gut milieu stands poised as a potential modulator in the mitigation of inflammatory surges.

Dietary fibre assumes a pivotal role in nurturing gut health, functioning as a nourishing medium for advantageous gut microflora. A bounty of fibrous-rich edibles, encompassing fruits, vegetables, whole grains, legumes, and nuts, are reliable sources of fibre. Aide to this, prebiotics, characterised by their non-digestible nature, impart a stimulatory impetus to the proliferation and metabolic vigour of beneficial gut microorganisms.

Prominent examples of prebiotic-rich foods include garlic, onions, leeks, asparagus, bananas, and oats, offering commendable reservoirs of biologically active fibres. Additionally, probiotics are beneficial bacteria that can be ingested through fermented foods or supplements. They help to regenerate and maintain a healthy gut microbiome. Fermented foods like yogurt, kefir, sauerkraut, kimchi, miso, and tempeh are good sources of probiotics.

Polyphenols, which are bioactive constituents sourced from plants, exhibit antioxidative and anti-inflammatory attributes. Their potential contribution to strengthening gut health stems from their capacity to engender a favourable habitat for the proliferation of advantageous microflora. Good sources of polyphenols encompass edibles like berries, cocoa, green tea, and olive oil, distinguished for their rich polyphenolic content.

Fermented foods undergo a natural transformative process whereby salubrious microorganisms metabolise sugars into acids. This metabolic conversion not only imparts probiotic enrichment but also extends the prospect of supplementary health advantages. The incorporation of fermented nourishment within dietary regimens serves to bolster the vitality of the gut microbiome and expedite the mechanisms of proficient digestion.

Ensuring adequate hydration levels is a fundamental prerequisite for the promotion of gut health. The ingestion of a suitable volume of water plays a critical role in the preservation of the gut's mucosal lining, thereby bolstering the mechanisms of digestion. Furthermore, foods abundant in water content, such as cucumbers, watermelon, and celery, extend a contributory role in both hydration and the fostering of digestive well-being.

The cultivation of dietary diversity is a pivotal tenet in fostering gut health, facilitating the provision of an array of nutrients and the promotion of a heterogeneous gut microbiome. Practicing moderation in dietary selections, particularly with respect to the consumption of processed foods, saccharine commodities, and deleterious fats, is a prudent strategy in the pursuit of sustaining gut health and overall holistic wellness.

Undoubtedly, gut health occupies a salient echelon within the paradigm of comprehensive well-being, casting its influence across spheres encompassing digestion, immune competence, psychological equilibrium, and the modulation of inflammatory responses.

The prevalence of heavily processed and fast foods in contemporary dietary patterns has surged due to their widespread availability and cost-effectiveness. Nevertheless, these culinary options typically offer scant essential nutrients while boasting elevated levels of detrimental components. Consistent consumption of such food can give rise to a host of undesirable health vulnerabilities and foster the progression of enduring heath conditions. These edibles tend to carry a surplus of calories, injurious fats, processed sugars, and sodium, while concurrently lacking in vital nutrients such as vitamins, minerals, and dietary fibre.

Consistently indulging in fast and heavily processed foods can result in deficiencies in essential nutrients, as they lack the vital elements necessary for optimal well-being. Since these foods tend to be dense in calories but are lacking in essential nutrients, it will result in a surplus of calories ingested without satisfying one's appetite.

The excessive consumption of unfavourable fats and added sugars can precipitate weight gain, elevating the vulnerability to obesity, an eminent forerunner to a gamut of chronic ailments such as cardiovascular disorders, diabetes, and specific cancers.

High sodium content in processed and fast foods can aid the development of high blood pressure or hypertension, which is a considerable risk factor for heart disease. Frequently consuming heavily processed and fast foods, specifically those high in added sugars and refined carbohydrates, can result in insulin resistance and a heightened risk of developing type 2 diabetes. These foods are typically low in fibre, which is fundamental for healthy digestion. A diet low in fibre can lead to constipation and other digestive problems.

Certain processed foods can harbour additives, preservatives, and chemical compounds that have been correlated with an elevated susceptibility to specific forms of cancer. Diets rich in processed meats, encompassing items like hot dogs, bacon, and deli selections, have demonstrated an augmented likelihood of colorectal cancer occurrence. Furthermore, a discernible association exists between diets dominated by heavily processed and fast foods and an amplified propensity for experiencing depressive and anxious states.

.

The insufficiency of essential nutrients alongside the consumption of deleterious fats and sugars can exert adverse effects on both cerebral health and emotional well-being. It is noteworthy that heavily processed edibles are frequently meticulously engineered to elicit heightened palatability, potentially culminating in compulsive eating behaviours and injurious cravings.

These food items have the capacity to supersede innate hunger cues, thereby contributing to excessive consumption and instigating a cycle characterised by suboptimal dietary selections. An array of heavily processed and fast foods is predisposed to fostering bodily inflammation, a phenomenon intrinsically correlated with a spectrum of enduring ailments, including arthritis, cardiovascular maladies, and diabetes. The allure of convenience and accessibility that accompanies heavily processed and fast foods is counterbalanced by their substantial health ramifications.

Regular indulgence in these foods can culminate in inadequate nutritional intake, obesity, cardiovascular disorders, diabetes, gastrointestinal complications, and an elevated susceptibility to specific diseases. Beyond these physical implications, their impact extends to mental well-being, as they have the potential to instigate food dependencies and yearnings, while concurrently propagating inflammatory processes within the body.

To bolster general well-being and diminish the susceptibility to enduring ailments, it becomes imperative to afford precedence to nutrient-dense, unprocessed whole foods, while concurrently curtailing the consumption of heavily processed and fast foods. Embracing a well-rounded and diverse dietary regimen that encompasses an assortment of fruits, vegetables, whole grains, lean protein sources, and healthful fats can markedly enhance health outcomes and overall quality of life.

Sustainable and organic eating entails a nutritional strategy that encompasses not solely personal well-being but also the repercussions of dietary selections on the ecosystem, biodiversity, and forthcoming generations. This approach underscores a synergistic correlation between human welfare and the global environment.

The ethos of sustainable and organic eating champions agricultural methodologies that foster soil vitality, mitigate pollution, and safeguard water reservoirs. Through organic farming, the utilisation of synthetic pesticides, herbicides, and genetically modified organisms (GMOs) is avoided, thereby averting potential harm to wildlife and soil microorganisms.

Opting for foods sourced through sustainable means allows individuals to play a role in safeguarding natural habitats and bolstering biodiversity. Industrial agriculture, including the production of heavily processed foods, significantly contributes to greenhouse gas emissions and climate change. Contrarily, sustainable, and organic farming practices often exhibit diminished carbon footprints and the potential to isolate carbon dioxide within the soil, thereby contributing to climate change mitigation efforts.

Organic produce is cultivated devoid of synthetic chemicals, potentially mitigating the risk of exposure to deleterious residues, and fostering enduring well-being. The paradigm of sustainable and organic eating accentuates the consumption of whole, nutrient-dense foods, emblematic of their intrinsic advantages for overall health and the prevention of ailments.

Sustainable and organic farming practices advocate for the conservation of traditional and heirloom crop strains, contributing to the preservation of agricultural diversity and fortification against pests and diseases. Opting for locally procured, sustainably generated foods not only support local farmers and economies but also cultivates community bonds while concurrently mitigating the carbon emissions linked to extensive transportation distances.

Embracing sustainable eating practices entails fostering a conscientious awareness of food selections and restricting food wastage. This concerted effort serves to conserve valuable resources and limit the ecological ramifications stemming from food creation and disposal.

Organic and sustainable farming practices typically prioritise the humane treatment of animals, providing them with adequate space, access to the outdoors, and natural diets. Sustainable agricultural practices, like crop rotation and agroforestry, can improve soil fertility and resilience, contributing to long-term food security in a changing climate.

Adopting sustainable and organic eating practices nurtures an understanding of the pivotal role that deliberate dietary selections play in shaping both the environment and the prospects of succeeding generations. This approach spurs individuals to cultivate a heightened awareness of diverse food production systems and to champion policies that reinforce sustainable methodologies.

Anchored in a comprehensive perspective on well-being, sustainable and organic eating recognises the intrinsic interdependence of human health, the environment, and the global community. Beyond being a mere dietary preference, this ethos encapsulates a conscientious and ethical stance towards food consumption, one that steadfastly considers the welfare of the planet, its ecosystems, and the well-being of forthcoming generations.

Embracing a lifelong commitment to healthy eating entails the necessity of strategizing your meals for the week ahead and devising a corresponding shopping list. This proactive approach aids in maintaining focus and deters unplanned procurement of unwholesome products. It is advisable to avoid grocery shopping on an empty stomach, as such a scenario can inadvertently trigger impulsive acquisition of calorie-laden food and unhealthy snacks.

Check the nutrition labels of packaged foods to make informed choices. Look for items with lower amounts of saturated fats, added sugars, and sodium. Choose whole, unprocessed foods whenever possible. Pick out whole grains, fresh fruits and vegetables, and lean proteins like poultry, fish, and beans. Go for hydration choices like water, herbal teas, or alternatives with lower calorie content, rather than sugary beverages.

When navigating the store, sidestep aisles housing sugary snacks and processed indulgences. Aim to curtail purchases of heavily processed fare such as chips, cookies, and pre-packaged meals, which often carry an excess of harmful fats, added sugars, and sodium. Prioritise stocking up on nourishing snacks like fresh fruits, sliced vegetables, nuts, or low-fat yogurt for swift and healthful selections. Consider opting for smaller portions of certain items like snacks or treats, enjoying them in moderation.

Whenever feasible, opt for locally sourced and seasonal produce. Not only does this choice ensure freshness, but it also extends support to local farmers while mitigating the environmental footprint of long-distance transportation. In your quest for the best selections aligned with your budget and health, take the time to compare prices and nutritional content across various brands.

Allocating ample time for your shopping trip is crucial to avoiding hasty decisions driven by pressure. Shopping under duress can potentially lead to impulsive choices that are not in line with your health goals.

Explore novel fruits, vegetables, whole grains, or healthful recipes to introduce variety into your culinary repertoire. This diversified approach to your diet can render the pursuit of healthy eating a more gratifying and sustainable endeavour. Direct your attention towards food that offer a substantial wealth of nutrients in relation to their calorie content.

Opting for items characterised by high nutrient density augments their positive impact on well-being. By integrating these strategies into your routine while shopping, you can actively steer your dietary choices towards healthier options and uphold your commitment to nutritious eating objectives.

By nurturing mindfulness in your choices, you empower yourself to compose a grocery cart that resonates with balance and nutrition. It's important to acknowledge that the journey of healthy eating is ongoing, and an occasional indulgence in treats is acceptable if it's balanced by a broader focus on predominantly wholesome choices.

Embrace cooking techniques that prioritise your well-being, such as baking, grilling, steaming, or roasting, as opposed to frying. These methods necessitate less additional fat and better preserve the nutritional value of food. Employ salt judiciously in your culinary endeavours, and elevate taste by incorporating herbs, spices, and natural flavourings. Infuse your meals with vibrantly coloured fruits and vegetables, as each colour signifies a distinct medley of nutrients.

Chart a course for nutritional balance by premeditating your meals in advance, thus ensuring comprehensive nourishment throughout the week. Streamline your culinary process by preparing and portioning ingredients ahead of time, facilitating swift and uncomplicated assembly on busier days. Prioritise lean protein sources, such as skinless poultry, fish, tofu, beans, and legumes, all of which possess reduced levels of saturated fats and contribute to cardiovascular wellness.

Incorporate nourishing fat sources, such as avocados, nuts, seeds, and olive oil, into your meals. These healthy fats contribute to cognitive well-being and facilitate the absorption of fat-soluble vitamins. Ensure that vegetables are cooked to a tender-crisp state, preserving both their inherent nutrients and their innate flavours. Efficiently utilise leftovers by transforming them into novel dishes, thus curtailing food wastage and streamlining your culinary experience.

Exercise discernment when perusing recipes and contemplate potential adjustments to diminish the presence of added sugars, detrimental fats, and excessive salt. Whenever feasible, make substitutions with more healthful ingredients. Encourage family members to participate in meal planning and preparation. This fosters a sense of ownership and makes mealtime enjoyable for everyone.

Embark on culinary adventures by delving into recipes hailing from various cultures. This exploration opens doors to unfamiliar ingredients and cooking methodologies that contribute to a diet abundant in diversity and nourishment. Prioritise adherence to established food safety protocols to avert the risk of foodborne ailments. Adhere to the principles of cleanliness, segregation, thorough cooking, and proper refrigeration.

Healthy cooking is a powerful proficiency that enables you to take control of nutrition and to make choices that fosters overall well-being. By using whole, fresh ingredients, choosing healthy cooking methods, and being mindful of portion sizes, you can create nutritious and delicious meals.

Mindful eating constitutes a disciplined practice characterised by undivided focus on the act of consuming, free from judgment or distraction. This approach entails wholehearted engagement with the present, relishing the intricacies of flavours and texture inherent in food, while simultaneously cultivating an awareness of signals for hunger and satiety. Beyond mere nutrition, mindful eating transcends to encompass the complete experience of dining and its profound impact on overall well-being.

It advocates unhurried and purposeful consumption, thereby elevating the efficacy of the digestive process. The thorough mastication of food aids in fostering proper digestion and optimal absorption of nutrients. By attuning to one's hunger and fullness cues, mindful eating emerges as a preventative measure against overindulgence, actively bolstering the management of a healthy weight.

Mindful eating facilitates an enhanced recognition of triggers tied to emotional eating, paving the way for the cultivation of healthier strategies to manage stress and emotional responses. It also engenders a heightened affinity with the nourishment we consume, generating a more profound acknowledgment of its origin and the labour invested in its preparation.

Deliberately dedicating time to relishing the intricacies of flavours, fragrance, and texture accentuates the allure of the culinary journey.

By maintaining mindfulness concerning dietary choices and eating habits, individuals can mitigate the inclination toward impulsive consumption, binge eating, and detrimental cravings. The practice of mindful eating consequently contributes to augmenting mental well-being, fostering a constructive rapport with food, and nurturing a positive body image.

Paying attention to the sensory facets of eating augments the pleasure derived from meals, which contributes to a more satisfying eating experience. Mindful eating enables individuals to enjoy occasional treats or indulgent foods while being mindful of portion sizes and overall dietary balance.

By being fully present during meals, individuals can nurture a deeper connection to food, improve digestion, and enhance overall well-being. Mindful eating is more than just about the nutritional aspects of food, it promotes a positive relationship with eating, supports mental and emotional health, and fosters a holistic approach to well-being. Incorporating mindful eating into daily life can lead to numerous benefits that extend beyond physical health, contributing to a more balanced and satisfying relationship with food and the body.

Healthy eating surpasses a transient dietary regimen. It constitutes an enduring way of life cantered around nourishing the body with foods rich in nutrients and cultivating thoughtful dietary decisions. Emphasising the perspective of healthy eating as a sustainable lifestyle, rather than a transitory regimen, stands as a pivotal component in realising lasting health and holistic welfare.

Adopting healthy eating as an enduring lifestyle yields continuous and viable health advantages. This approach fosters comprehensive well-being, curtails susceptibility to chronic ailments, and amplifies longevity. Conversely, brief diets often result in short-lived weight loss, frequently followed by weight regain once the regimen concludes. In contrast, embracing healthy eating as a lifestyle promotes for an enduring approach to weight management, devoid of extreme restrictions or drastic transformations.

Incorporating healthy eating into one's lifestyle fosters the cultivation of mindful and intuitive dietary practices. Individuals acquire the skill of attuning to their bodies, heeding signals of hunger and fullness, and making educated decisions regarding nourishment.

A healthy eating lifestyle centres around the provision of essential nutrients to the body, ensuring a supply of crucial vitamins, minerals, and macronutrients for optimal performance. This comprehensive approach resonates with enhanced mental health and emotional well-being. A well-rounded diet can alleviate stress, anxiety, and depression, cultivating a positive outlook.

The integration of healthy eating as a lifestyle encourages sustained behavioural transformation. It necessitates the forging of novel habits and attitudes toward food that seamlessly embed into everyday existence. Anchored in the principles of enjoyment and sustainability, a healthy eating lifestyle permits occasional indulgences while upholding a balanced and nutritious dietary pattern.

Incorporating healthy eating into one's daily life possesses the power to ignite inspiration and exert a favourable impact on those around them, including family and friends, propelling them toward the adoption of corresponding practices. The bedrock of a healthy eating lifestyle rests upon the accentuation of enduring health objectives. It impels individuals to accord precedence to their well-being across the expanse of time.

The embrace of a healthy eating lifestyle engenders a harmonious rapport with food, unburdened by feelings of guilt or the constraints of rigid regulations. Often synonymous with judicious food choices, the principles of a healthy eating lifestyle resonate with the ideals of sustainability, underpinning endeavours in environmental preservation and a reduction in carbon footprint.

Wholeheartedly adopting healthy eating as a lifestyle, rather than a transitory dietary phase, stands as an imperative in the pursuit of enduring health advantages, the maintenance of sustainable weight, and the augmentation of overall well-being. The ethos of a healthy eating lifestyle extends its influence to fostering favourable mental health, endorsing the practice of intuitive eating, and affording the liberty to make diversified dietary choices.

Through the embrace of healthy eating as an unwavering commitment throughout one's existence, individuals are poised to unlock an elevated standard of living, savour positive associations with nourishment, and kindle a beacon that beckons others to similarly prioritise their health and wellness.

Chapter 5 - The Role of Physical Activity on Longevity

In an era where the pursuit of a longer and healthier life has captured our collective imagination, the sophisticated relationship between lifestyle choices and longevity has become a subject of intense scrutiny. Among these lifestyle factors, physical activity stands as a beacon of promise, offering a multifaceted approach to enhancing both the quantity and quality of years lived. The age-old adage "move it or lose it" takes on new significance as scientific research consistently unveils the remarkable impact of exercise on ageing and longevity.

As we embark on a journey into the fascinating nexus between physical activity and longevity, it becomes important to delve beyond the surface benefits of exercise to uncover the elaborate cellular mechanisms, hormonal adaptations, and profound physiological changes that contribute to extending human lifespan. We will explore the insightful effects of exercise on cardiovascular health, metabolic balance, cognitive function, immune resilience, and the delicate balance between our bodies and longevity.

In this exploration, we will journey through the scientific considerations that illuminate the links between exercise and cellular rejuvenation, plaiting a tapestry of insight that underscores how movement isn't just an accessory to life but a catalyst for its preservation.

From the microcosm of DNA telomeres to the macroscopic domains of heart health and bone density, the story of exercise and longevity unfetters in a work of health span extension.

Physical activity, the art of harmonising body and motion, entails a vast spectrum of exertions. From our everyday movements to the structured paces of a fitness regimen, it is a journey towards vitality and well-being. Regular engagement in these motile endeavours confers a treasure trove of health benefits, revealing the path to enduring wellness.

Among these movements, the ballet of aerobic exercises takes centre stage, coordinating an opus of heartbeats and breaths. There's the graceful tango of walking, accessible in almost any corner of our world. For those who seek a more fervent tempo, running and jogging offer climaxes of cardiovascular rewards. Cycling, whether in the open air or on the steady pulse of a stationary bike, brings a rhythm of lower-body endurance.

And in the liquid embrace of water, swimming schemes a full-body workout, kind to the joints, soothingly buoyant. The significance of strength training reverberates, as muscles awaken and fortify through the resistance of weights and the weight of our own bodies. Weightlifting, with its iron instruments of transformation, encompasses squats, bench presses, and arm curls. Bodyweight exercises, a testament to our own physical potential, conjure strength from push-ups, squats, and planks.

Within the realm of flexibility and mobility, the rhythm of stretching resonates like a melody, expanding the boundaries of our movements and serving as a guardian against potential injuries. The time-honoured discipline of yoga intricately textures together postures, mindful breaths, and serene meditation, creating a rich embroidery of physical coordination and mental peace.

Nevertheless, it is the often-overlooked elements of equilibrium and steadiness that become indispensable, especially as the graceful years pass us by. Tai Chi is another practise to consider. It diligently hones our equilibrium, fortitude, and inner tranquillity, helping to harmonise the symmetries of our physical well-being with the grace of time's passage.

For those who seek an increase in pace, there's the dynamic tempo of High-Intensity Interval Training (HIIT), where intensity ignites calorie-burning flames. CrossFit, the high-intensity maestro, combines cardio and strength, while plyometrics incorporates power and coordination. With group fitness classes, structure meets motivation and social connection. Spinning or indoor cycling helps to elevate cardiovascular endurance. Hiking leads a spirited trek, engaging important muscles.

Kayaking and canoeing summon the upper-body serenade, a waterborne ballet of strength and coordination. Select your movement wisely, harmonising it with your fitness, goals, and passions. The ensemble of diverse physical activities crafts a well-rounded combination, with crescendos in cardiovascular health, muscular strength, flexibility, and mental serenity. A word of caution, tread carefully and seek counsel from healthcare professionals before embarking on this odyssey, especially if you bear the weight of pre-existing health concerns.

The perennial practice of physical activity extends our sojourn through life's narrative, as it generously influences an intricate interplay of physiological, psychological, and systemic processes within our mortal vessel. This manifold effect assumes the mantle of a guardian, shepherding us toward the realms of enduring health and longevity.

Our diligent engagement in physical activity becomes a marvel, guiding the heart and nurturing the cardiovascular system. Its melodies of movement yield a symphony of benefits that echo through the corridors of longevity.

Regular physical activity breathes vitality into the heart, endowing it with the grace to pump blood with the utmost efficiency. This enhancement fosters superior circulation and stands as a stalwart guardian against the spectre of heart disease. The heart, akin to a virtuoso, fine-tunes its rhythm, ensuring that each beat resounds with precision. Such mastery not only refines circulation but also forms an indomitable bulwark against the encroachments of cardiovascular maladies.

With each pulsation, we march towards a longer, healthier existence, where the shadows of heart ailments recede. In this elegant ballet of physicality, the heart takes centre stage, its cadence a testament to the wondrous interplay between effort and longevity.

Physical activity orchestrates a harmonious balance within the body, conducting a beautiful arrangement of health benefits that pulsate through our mortal coil. This choreography includes a series of essential movements, each contributing to the opus of a longer, healthier life. With each step, every exertion, physical activity takes on the role of a skilled conductor, maintaining the delicate tempo of our blood pressure. It skilfully lowers the risk of hypertension and the looming spectre of its complications.

Like a virtuoso with a finely tuned instrument, exercise plays a tune that elevates the levels of "good" HDL cholesterol while lowering the "bad" LDL cholesterol, preventing the discord of atherosclerosis from taking root. In the elegant dance of maintaining body weight, physical activity leads with grace and poise, preventing the encroachment of obesity and its entourage of health concerns.

Through the rhythmic expenditure of calories, it orchestrates weight loss and guards against the creeping gain. This metabolic disco, executed with precision, ensures a harmonious equilibrium in our body's metabolic orchestra. With increased muscle mass, it conducts a symphony of a heightened metabolic rate, facilitating the maintenance of a healthy weight and contributing to our journey toward longevity.

The regimen of regular exercise unfolds a cascade of benefits that tenderly cradle our well-being. As we traverse this path of vitality, we find that its influence extends into diverse realms of health creating harmonious outcomes. Within the domain of metabolic proficiency, regular exercise acts as an expert, tuning the body's response to insulin with precision. This modulation composes a reduction in the perilous shadows of type 2 diabetes, enhancing our prospects for enduring health.

In the rhythmic balance of regulation, physical activity assumes the role of choreographer, ensuring that blood sugar levels pirouette gracefully within the safe bounds of health. With each step and every movement, it gently escorts us away from the precipice of diabetes-related complications.

The body, under the careful tutelage of physical activity, embarks on an elegant pas de deux between bone and muscle. Engaging in weight-bearing exercises and strength training ensures this duet resonates with harmony. Weight-bearing activities and resistance training foster the enduring strength of our bones.

This safeguarding reduces the looming spectre of osteoporosis and the fractures it may beckon. Strength training, much like a vigilant guardian, thwarts the incursions of age-related muscle loss known as sarcopenia. This vigilant protection not only bolsters our overall functional capacity but also unfurls a defence against the perils of falls.

In the ethereal realm of the mind, regular physical activity serenades our brain health and cognitive prowess. It unfurls a rhapsody of benefits, enhancing the very essence of our mental faculties. Physical activity, as a conductor of circulation, coordinates an augmentation of blood flow to the brain. This nourishing cataract delivers the essential nutrients and oxygen required for sustained cognitive vitality.

Our cerebral landscape, under the tender touch of regular exercise, becomes a canvas for the masterpiece of neuroplasticity. This artistry of adaptability fortifies the citadels of learning and memory, harmonising our cognitive function. In the grand composition of our health and well-being, regular exercise takes centre stage, conducting a resonant opus that spans the spectrum of our physical and mental flourishing. Each note, each movement, each engagement in this composition extends an invitation to a life of enduring vitality.

The presence of chronic inflammation looms ominously, its connection to age related maladies undeniable. Yet, in physical activity, we unearth a profound ally in the quest to quell this silent adversary. The insidious link between chronic inflammation and a multitude of age-related afflictions is well-established.

Physical activity emerges as a vigilant scout, offering a measure of control over this unwelcome inflammation. Regular exercise coordinates a reduction in chronic low-grade inflammation, a quiet but persistent companion in chronic ailments. Its steady cadence harmonises with the rhythms of our body, silencing the discord of inflammation.

Physical activity plays a significant role in hormonal balance, regulating the integration of overall health and the ageing process. Its wand guiding hormonal harmony, leaving a profound impact on our very essence. Exercise prompts a variety of hormones, including the mood-lifting endorphins. This enriches the canvas of our well-being, infusing it with vibrant shades of vitality.

Within cellular processes, exercise is instrumental, influencing the intricate processes of ageing. It nurtures the well-being of our cellular powerhouses, known as mitochondria, enhancing the graceful energy ballet performed within our cells.

As we traverse the landscape of physical activity, we come to understand it not only as a promoter of physical fitness but also as an architect of holistic health. Its enduring influence extends from inflammation control and hormonal balance to the intricate details of our cellular processes. Thus, it beckons us towards a life characterised not only by longevity but also by vitality and well-being in every step we take.

Certainly, the cardiovascular advantages bestowed by consistent physical activity are profound, assuming a pivotal role in championing heart health and mitigating the peril of heart disease. These advantages encompass an array of physiological enhancements that collectively pave the way to a lengthier and more robust existence.

Through regular physical exertion, the heart muscle fortifies and refines its proficiency in propelling blood throughout the entire body. This in turn, begets a multitude of favourable consequences.

The volume of blood expelled with each heartbeat, known as stroke volume, surges with the engagement of exercise. Consequently, this mitigates the heart's workload, rendering it more adept in its function. Moreover, habitual exercise has the capacity to reduce your resting heart rate, emblematic of a more adept heart that labours less during periods of repose.

Physical activity, in its manifold virtues, serves as a catalyst for enhanced blood circulation, ensuring the efficient conveyance of life-sustaining oxygen and vital nutrients to every nook and cranny of the body, even tending to the heart's own needs.

Exercise helps orchestrate the expansion of blood vessels, a phenomenon known as vasodilation, thus augmenting the river of vitality coursing through our veins while reducing the looming gamut of obstructions. In this improved circulation, the risk of portentous blood clots is conspicuously diminished, their threat to heart and mind receding like distant echoes.

Regular engagement in exercise, a steadfast custodian, maintains the sentry of blood pressure at healthy ramparts, thereby warding off the perils of hypertension and its attendant tribulations. Exercise assumes the role of an alchemist, conjuring an elevation in the levels of high-density lipoprotein (HDL) cholesterol, often dubbed the "good" cholesterol.

This noble element embarks on a mission to expel excess cholesterol from the arterial highways, leaving them unburdened and open to the flow of life.

Exercise, that venerable ally of well-being, wields the power to drive down the levels of low-density lipoprotein (LDL) cholesterol, that notorious antagonist responsible for the insidious build-up of arterial plaque. Yet, its influence extends beyond the cholesterol ledger.

Within the intricate spheres of our circulatory system, endothelial cells assume the facade of protectors, guarding the inner sanctums of our blood vessels. They oversee a symphony of circulatory excellence, and regular exercise, it seems, is their favourite tune. With each workout, they don their finest performance, ensuring their proper function.

Healthy endothelial cells, in their prime, expand the crimson pathways, allowing for proper capillary dilation. This extension staves off the relentless grip of vessel constriction and bestows upon them a lasting flexibility. But exercise, in its wisdom, addresses another foe on the battlefield of heart health which is obesity. It seeks out visceral fat, the clandestine marauder lurking around our vital organs, a harbinger of heart disease and metabolic turmoil. With each stride and lift, exercise takes aim, diminishing this peril and safeguarding our cardiovascular well-being.

Physical activity stands as a cornerstone within the orbit of cardiac rehabilitation, extending its caring embrace to those who have weathered heart-related trials. In the aftermath of heart surgeries or cardiac setbacks, exercise programs emerge as stalwart allies, guiding patients along the path to recovery while nurturing the garden of their cardiovascular well-being.

Within the complex territory of heart health, there exists a delicate thread known as Heart Rate Variability (HRV), a sentinel of the heart's resilience and adaptability. Here, physical activity takes on the role of an artisan, adorning this thread with newfound lustre. As the pulse quickens with exercise, so too does the heart's concerto, harmonising with the rhythms of HRV. Together, they paint a picture of a balanced and vibrant autonomic nervous system, one that has been fortified and tuned by the artistry of physical activity.

In the grand orchestration of our physical well-being, the role of physical activity is nothing short of a miracle. It wields a substantial influence over our metabolism, weight management, and the critical endeavour of impeding obesity. These aspects are intricately connected, with each element contributing harmoniously to the overall composition of health and longevity.

Metabolism, the complex interplay of chemical reactions that sustains life, resides at the core of this narrative. It embodies the transformative essence within, turning nourishment into the vital energy that propels all our undertakings. In this context, physical activity emerges as a catalyst for transformation, coordinating metabolic adjustments with precision.

Consider, for instance, the effect of regular exercise, particularly the artistry of strength training. It confers upon us the gift of increased muscle mass, a transformation that reverberates throughout our metabolic ensemble. Muscles, with their vibrant activity, emerge as savant performers, consuming calories even when the curtains of rest have descended. This crescendo in resting metabolic rate organises more efficient energy utilisation, ensuring that the body becomes a skilled composer of its own health and vitality.

The energy expended during exercise is a vital contributor to our metabolism. The intensity of our physical exertion dictates the magnitude of energy consumed, both during the activity and in the post-workout aftermath. In this intricate metabolic mechanism, exercise dons yet another role, that of a maestro elevating the body's sensitivity to insulin.

Insulin, the guardian of blood sugar equilibrium, takes centre stage. With exercise's guidance, it sharpens its sensitivity, orchestrating a smoother performance in regulating blood sugar levels. This enhancement of insulin sensitivity becomes a bastion against the looming threats of insulin resistance and the onset of type 2 diabetes.

Delving into the space of physical exertion is akin to setting ablaze the caloric reserves, a phenomenon that transpires when paired harmoniously with a well-rounded dietary regimen. This equilibrium gives rise to a pivotal entity in weight management, the caloric deficit.

Exercise regimen, embraced diligently, bears the onus of safeguarding and sculpting the sacred edifices of lean muscle mass, all while ushering away the burdens of superfluous adiposity. In this transformation, a more gracious body composition emerges, like a sculptor chiselling away excess stone to reveal the exquisite form within flesh and spirit.

As this interplay between physical exertion and nutrition unfolds, the body's very essence undergoes a subtle metamorphosis. A delicate balance emerges, a tuneful ratio between muscle and fat. Physicality coaches the body to become an expert in the art of fat utilisation. Stored fat, once dormant, now ascends to stardom as the primary fuel, propelling the human engine with newfound vigour and efficiency. But the allure of exercise does not stop at the stage of bodily transformation, it extends its influence on the very domain of appetite.

The rhythmic cadence of physical activity orchestrates the harmony of hormones, a symphony that strives to bring equilibrium. Cravings, those capricious gustatory desires, find themselves tempered by this diligent maestro, and the impulse for excess sustenance bows in deference to a wiser, more measured indulgence.

Obesity, a multifaceted condition marked by the unwelcome accumulation of surplus body fat, unfurls a web of health intricacies, casting shadows over well-being. Amid this warren of challenges, the stalwart champion emerges, regular physical engagement, a formidable guardian against the encroaching spectre of obesity. This dynamic alliance between movement and well-being pivots upon the delicate equilibrium of energy, the sum of calories ingested, and calories expended. When this balance finds its tempo, the peril of obesity recedes.

A habitual embrace of physicality ensures that excess calories meet a fate far nobler than storage. They metamorphose into the very essence of vitality, fuelling the body's relentless journey. Within this accordant ballet, the maestros are the hormones orchestrating metabolism, particularly insulin and leptin. Exercise, the silent conductor, guides these hormonal symphonies, steering them away from discord and imbalance. Thus, the ominous shadow of obesity retreats, yielding ground to a brighter, more vibrant ensemble of health and vitality.

In the intricate spheres of well-being, the art of physical activity emerges as a potent shield against the encroachment of metabolic syndromes. This formidable cluster of conditions, characterised by the worrying presence of elevated blood pressure, heightened blood sugar, the unwelcome embrace of excess waistline fat, and the discord of abnormal cholesterol levels, casts a foreboding shadow over one's health landscape. In its wake, it ushers forth a congregation of perils, a cohort of maladies that find their roots in the realm of obesity.

Yet, with regular exercise, a transformative alchemy unfolds. It bequeaths unto us a luminous spectrum of emotional well-being, elevating mood and dissolving the tempestuous clouds of stress. In this sanctuary of movement, emotional eating finds its quietus, its siren call diminished. Thus, the path to obesity prevention is not only a physical journey but a song of heart and mind, harmonising to craft a healthier, more resilient self.

In the grand conduction of vitality, physical activity takes centre stage, supervising the mechanisms that safeguard the complex structures of bone density and muscle mass, two pillars of enduring health and functional harmony. As the sands of time sweep us into the embrace of ageing, nature's gentle hand ushers in a natural diminuendo of vital elements within our musculoskeletal repertoire. Yet, the gift of regular exercise emerges as the expert, bidding this decline to linger and bestowing upon us the flair of preservation.

When we engage in movement, where footsteps become the notes of a graceful composition, a cascade of benefits unfurls. Activities that bestow the weight of the world upon our bones, like stately walks, spirited jogs, and the rhythmic sway of dance, call forth the diligent artisans known as osteoblasts. These miniature architects of the skeletal system lay the foundation of resilience, building fresh bone tissue and nurturing the construction of heightened bone density. In this delicate interplay, we find the tone of renewal and the artistry of longevity.

In the arena of physical fitness, the artistry of strength training and resistance exercises, from the iron embrace of weightlifting to the subtle tension of resistance bands and the body's own resistance, offer a profound gift to our skeletal architecture. They bestow upon our bones a delicate yet invigorating gift, a ballet of stress and resilience.

This stress, far from being a foe, is a catalyst for transformation. It whispers to the bones, beckoning them to evolve, to fortify their essence. In response, our bones embark on a journey of adaptation, growing denser and mightier, like seasoned sentinels of our inner fortress.

With each exertion, a composition of growth factors is summoned, nurturing the very essence of bone health. The theatre of physical stress, set upon the stage of our activities, unfurls a process of renewal akin to an artist's brush strokes on a canvas. Old bone tissue gracefully yields to the emergence of new, robust layers, renewing the very tapestry of our skeletal strength. Thus, we fortify our citadels, rendering them resilient and less susceptible to the fractures of time.

In the area of mindful movement, certain activities, like the pulsing dance of jumping and the dynamic artistry of plyometric exercises, emerge as benevolent sculptors of our skeletal strength. They navigate the delicate balance between exertion and care, extending a graceful invitation to our bones for a harmonious sway of rejuvenation.

With each calculated impact, the stage is set for transformation. These deliberate encounters with force, while seemingly daunting, beget a profound gift, the generation of micro-fractures that serve as the harbingers of change. In response to these subtle fissures, our bones orchestrate a mechanism of growth and repair, becoming sturdier and more resilient.

In parallel, the theatre of weight-bearing exercises unfolds, where calcium takes centre stage. This essential mineral, a cornerstone of bone health, finds its role magnified in the presence of physicality. As for the grand maestro of muscle maintenance, strength training ascends to the podium. It calls forth our muscle fibres, compelling them to adapt and flourish in the face of resistance.

With this composition of effort, muscle atrophy, the ageing chameleon, retreats into the shadows. In its place, we bear witness to the enduring vitality of muscle and the grace of a body in harmonious motion.

There exists a profound symphony conducted by the hand of physical activity, particularly the artistry of resistance training. This symphony resonates within the very heart of muscle cells, where the harmonious notes of protein synthesis are played. Here, within the quiet chambers of our muscle fibres, construction and repair unfolds, meticulously crafting and refurbishing the fabric of muscle tissue. It is a testament to the preservation of strength and endurance, the safeguarding of our bodily fortresses.

In this tango of exertion, hormones emerge as the experts, wielding their batons to evoke a crescendo of growth and maintenance. Testosterone and growth hormones, these skilful messengers, echo through the corridors of our biology, calling forth the mighty forces of muscle growth.

Yet, this extends beyond the confines of the gym or exercise studio. It reverberates in our daily lives, where we carry groceries, ascend stairs, and perform countless feats of strength and coordination. These everyday activities of effort serve as a continuous challenge to our muscles, fostering their resilience and tenacity. Through this, we orchestrate the timeless tale of muscle preservation, an ode to strength enduring.

The role of nutrition, especially the ample supply of proteins, emerges as a vital cornerstone in the maintenance of our muscular strength. Yet, the true strength unfolds when this nourishment harmonises with the cadence of exercise. A diverse array of exercises takes centre stage, each movement targets distinct muscle groups, fostering equilibrium and safeguarding the holistic health of our musculature.

Moreover, exercise serves as an instrumentalist, orchestrating a masterpiece of communication between our nervous system and muscles. It enhances the synergy between these vital components, facilitating the recruitment and harmonious function of our muscles. In this intricate interplay, strength and resilience find their crescendo.

In the flowing journey of ageing, the preservation of mobility and the prevention of age-related muscle decline emerge as pivotal facets. These elements, far from being mere afterthoughts, serve as the bedrock upon which a life of substance in later years is built. They wield profound influence, not only shaping the quality of our existence but also acting as vigilant watchmen against the presence of injury, while safeguarding the sacred realm of independence and holistic well-being.

Mobility, that elusive but invaluable gift, encapsulates the essence of the human spirit's kinetic potential. It embodies the capacity to traverse through existence, unhindered and unburdened. The maintenance of this treasured attribute bears profound significance, as it empowers individuals to execute the ordinary tasks of life with grace and self-sufficiency.

From the simplicity of a stroll to the grace of a bend, the reach of a hand, or the ascent from a chair, mobility breathes life into these quotidian feats, preserving the sanctity of functional independence. In doing so, it gifts older adults with the priceless ability to safeguard and sustain their cherished quality of life.

The diminishment of mobility within the older adult population serves as a potent harbinger of peril, amplifying the presence of life-altering falls. These unforeseen stumbles, while appearing innocuous, unfurl a tapestry of dire consequences, often culminating in injury-induced hospitalisations, debilitating fractures, and, tragically, the forfeiture of life itself.

In stark contrast, the preservation of one's mobility emerges as an ardent guardian, diligently shielding against the precipice of such misfortunes. Through this vigilant stewardship, individuals craftily bolster their equilibrium, coordination, and agility, thereby diligently whittling away the spectre of falls.

The virtuous cycle of regular movement, ever the ally, ensures that joints remain amply lubricated and nourished, standing as steadfast sentinels against the encroachment of stiffness, discomfort, and the debilitation wrought by conditions such as arthritis. In the quiet tempo of regular motion, blood courses steadily through the network of veins and arteries, nourishing extremities, and vital organs alike.

This ceaseless circulation, a testament to the body's resilience, develops a protective mantle against the ominous clouds of circulatory tribulations and the manifold complications they usher in. In sum, the preservation of mobility becomes not just a means to traverse the years but a pledge to safeguard one's physical autonomy and well-being against the vagaries of time.

Within the intricate complexities of our well-being, physical activity emerges as the ace, masterfully composing a performance deep within the recesses of our intestines. This rhythmic pulse of vitality weaves its verses into the sweeping epic of gastrointestinal health. Yet, the sway of mobility extends its influence beyond the corporeal realm, painting an intricate tableau of heightened mood and enhanced mental well-being, akin to the interplay of light and shadow upon a canvas.

The ability to traverse the world gracefully fosters not only a sense of autonomy but also bestows upon us a vibrant bouquet of accomplishments, each petal symbolising a victory over the encroaching constraints of ageing. In this dance of life, mobility, both physical and metaphorical, assumes the mantle of paramount importance.

In this liberating mobility, older adults discover a passport to participation in social soirées, cherished hobbies, and exploratory outings. These endeavours are more than mere pastimes, they form the nucleus of a robust social network, the bastion against the encroaching solitude that shadows us with age. Thus, the art of movement, both physical and metaphorical, emerges as a conductor of vitality, uniting the threads of health, joy, and human connection in the grand tapestry of life.

The silent thief of muscle, known as sarcopenia, stealthily saps our strength and vitality, diminishing the wellspring of our functional capacity. In the quest for graceful ageing, the prevention of sarcopenia emerges as a steadfast affiliate, empowering older adults to maintain their physical prowess and embrace life's richness to the fullest.

In this unfolding narrative, the significance of muscle strength takes centre stage. It serves as the bedrock upon which our balance and stability are erected, fortifying our defences against the perilous precipice of falls and their attendant injuries.

Beneath the surface, these muscular marvels consume the flames of calories at rest, far outstripping the modest appetite of their fat counterparts. The prevention of muscle loss thus not only safeguards physical prowess but also keeps the embers of our resting metabolic rate burning brightly. This, in turn, offers a potent tool in the management of body weight, warding off the invasions of obesity. In this interplay of strength and resilience, the prevention of muscle loss stands as a guardian of both physical and metabolic vigour, ensuring that the pages of ageing are penned with vitality and well-being.

Within our intricate physiology, muscles take the lead role, their elegant movements constructing an array of benefits that extend far beyond mere strength and motion. As they exert their force upon our bones during every movement, they become champions of bone health and density, the stalwart defenders against the threats of fractures and osteoporosis.

But their contributions don't end there. Muscle tissue emerges as an expert performer in the symphony of metabolic harmony, wielding its wand to regulate blood sugar levels with finesse. The prevention of muscle loss, therefore, stands as an ode to improved insulin sensitivity, a shield against the lurking shadow of type 2 diabetes.

Strong muscles grant older adults the autonomy to perform tasks independently, reducing reliance on others for assistance. With each flex, they script tales of endurance and stamina, allowing for the sustained engagement in activities without fatigue.

In the hidden alcoves of their cellular composition, muscles produce a treasury of substances, including myokines, which unfurl a range of anti-inflammatory and metabolic benefits, their contributions extending to the broader canvas of overall health. In this grand performance, muscles emerge as not just protagonists of movement but as architects of a life imbued with vitality and well-being.

Physical activity emerges as a resolute guardian against the encroaching shadows of cognitive decline and the formidable phantom of disorders like dementia. The brain, a marvel of nature, is far from static, it boasts a remarkable capacity for adaptation and change, a phenomenon we refer to as neuroplasticity.

Regular engagement in physical activity unfurls an array of virtues that unfailingly bolster brain health and amplify cognitive function. As we engage in physical activity, a steady surge of blood flows to our brains, a river of life that carries with it the precious cargo of essential nutrients and oxygen, nourishing the very essence of our cognitive function.

This improved circulation plays a dual role, not only fostering the vitality of brain cells but also serving as a diligent custodian, facilitating the efficient removal of waste products. But the story doesn't end there. With each stride and every push, physical activity becomes a maestro, orchestrating the release of neurotrophic factors, those remarkable proteins that serve as guardians of neuronal growth, survival, and overall well-being.

Among these aces, the brain-derived neurotrophic factor (BDNF) takes centre stage, its performance dedicated to nurturing the very cradle of our thoughts and memories, the neurons. In this narrative, physical activity emerges as not merely a means to sculpt the body but as a cherished partner in the eternal dance of the mind, a symphony conductor orchestrating the harmonious growth and preservation of our intellectual essence.

In the elaborate web of our biology, physical activity wields a profound influence over our neurotransmitters, those molecular messengers that design the intricate signals between neurons. In this masterpiece of science, exercise emerges as an instrumentalist, skilfully orchestrating the release of key neurotransmitters like dopamine and serotonin. These chemical experts, renowned for their roles in regulating mood and cognitive function, take centre stage in the auditorium of our minds.

But the saga doesn't conclude with neurotransmitters alone. Regular physical activity unfolds yet another chapter, one of defence against the looming spectres of oxidative stress and inflammation, both known culprits in the narrative of cognitive decline and the onset of neurodegenerative disorders. In this compelling narrative, reduced levels of oxidative stress and inflammation form the stalwart guardians of our precious brain cells, shielding them from the corrosive effects of damage.

Yet, there is more to this tale. Enter synaptic plasticity, the brain's wondrous capacity to craft new connections among neurons. Physical activity, in its wisdom, emerges as a devoted supporter of this synaptic environment, enabling the brain to adapt and reorganise its complex networks. The outcome is improved learning, enhanced memory, and heightened cognitive flexibility, a harmonious crescendo of mental competency.

In this narrative, physical activity transcends the realm of the body, becoming an esteemed expert, conducting the work of neurotransmitters and synaptic plasticity, crafting a sphere that resonates with improved mood, sharper cognition, and a vibrant, adaptable mind.

Physical activity wields profound influence over our well-being. It orchestrates a symphony of effects that resonate through our bodies and minds. In the realm of physiology, the act of moving our bodies triggers a wondrous alchemy. It fine-tunes our sensitivity to insulin, reigning in the capricious whims of blood sugar levels. This harmonious regulation stands as a bulwark against the perils of cognitive decline and the ominous spectre of Alzheimer's disease. Yet, the benefits extend far beyond the confines of the body.

As we engage in exercise, it is as if we enter a sanctuary of serenity, where stress and anxiety find no refuge. Our mental well-being blossoms like a resilient flower, as stress dissipates, so too does the fog that can obscure our cognitive faculties. The mind becomes sharper, more vibrant, and resilient. It is in these moments of physical exertion that we sow the seeds of a healthier brain, nurturing its growth.

Within the convolutions of the brain, grey matter thrives, expanding in regions associated with memory and learning. Meanwhile, the delicate drapery of white matter tracts, those silent messengers that facilitate communication between distant realms of thought, grows more robust. In every step, every heartbeat, and every movement, the journey towards a sound mind and a vibrant brain unfolds. In the domain of physical activity, the narrative of our well-being is written, chapter by chapter, in the remarkable story of our bodies and minds.

The rhythmic cadence of regular physical activity bestows upon us the gift of cardiovascular well-being, forging a shield against the encroaching shadows of afflictions such as hypertension and atherosclerosis. In the intricate interplay of our bodies, cardiovascular health emerges as the sentinel, its vitality intimately entwined with the sanctum of our minds.

For within the labyrinth of arteries and veins lies a profound connection to the inner altar of cognition. The blood, the vital river coursing through our vessels, is the life force that sustains not only our organs but the very essence of our thoughts. A robust and healthy cardiovascular system nourishes the brain, fuelling its faculties with the oxygen and nutrients necessary for peak performance.

In this magnificent orchestration of bodily and mental harmony, our actions play pivotal roles. When we engage in the pursuits of intellect and physical exertion, we become architects of cognitive reserve, a fortress of resilience. This remarkable phenomenon, wherein the brain fortifies itself against the ravages of time and circumstance, delays the inexorable march of cognitive decline and the spectre of neurodegenerative afflictions.

In the symphony of life, the confluence of movement, cognition, and cardiovascular vigour forms a triumvirate, crafting not only a healthier body but also a shielded sanctuary for our thoughts and memories. In the pursuit of wellness, we find ourselves as guardians of this precious equilibrium, nurturing our cardiovascular health to preserve the sanctity of our minds.

With regular physical activity, we unearth a treasure trove of psychological riches, each facet contributing to our mental well-being. It is a work of effects that reverberate through the corridors of our mind, forging a profound connection between the body's movements and our emotions and thoughts.

Exercise, that faithful companion of the active soul, wields a direct influence over the very chemistry of our brain. It orchestrates a harmonious interplay, finely tuning emotional equilibrium and enhancing cognitive prowess. As the heart quickens and muscles flex, stress retreats, mood elevates, and a profound sense of mental well-being takes root.

Elevated cortisol levels sound the alarm of the "fight or flight" response, casting shadows of anxiety and apprehension. Here, exercise emerges as the guardian of balance, ushering cortisol back to its rightful levels, ensuring that stress remains harmonious and in check.

In the pages of a life enriched by regular exercise, stress finds its antithesis, and mental well-being flourishes. The story of movement and its profound impact on our inner world unfolds, reminding us that the path to peace of mind is paved by the rhythm of our steps and the beat of our hearts.

.

The shadows of depression and anxiety are banished, as exercise, like a magician, conjures an elevated mood and dispels the spirit of sadness. In its wake, emotional well-being expands, vibrant and resplendent. Yet, the magic of physical activity extends beyond the chemistry of our minds. It is a sanctuary where the cacophony of stressors and negative thoughts fades into obscurity. Here, the body's graceful motions and precise coordination become the keys to mindfulness, offering respite from the relentless cycle of rumination.

In the crucible of this engagement, mental resilience is forged. It is an armour, a shield against the trials and tribulations that life may throw our way. With each step, each lift, and each stretch, we nurture the strength to navigate the challenges of existence with grace and composure.

In the quietude of movement, we discover the fortitude to face life's tempests head-on. In the monarchy of physical activity, the body and mind unite in a harmonious ballet, their partnership crafting an opus of joy, resilience, and serenity. It is a testament to the profound connection between motion and emotion, where the pursuit of health becomes the quest for inner harmony.

Embarking on the journey of attaining fitness objectives, whether they stand as towering peaks or modest hills, grants upon us a profound sense of accomplishment and self-mastery. In this domain of personal triumphs, our spirits are kindled, and the seeds of mental resilience take root.

With physical endeavour, the demands of exercise become a crucible for emotional stress. Here, amidst the pulsing beat of movement, we find an artful means to confront the tempest of difficult emotions and the trials of challenging circumstances. It becomes our sanctuary, a productive outlet for the inner turmoil we all must bear.

As we embrace the path of physical exertion, the very essence of our being undergoes transformation. The blood, coursing vigorously through our veins, carries with it the gift of enhanced cognition. The mind, invigorated by improved circulation, ascends to new heights of clarity and decision-making expertise.

And in this intricate mechanism, we find the antidote to the shadows that may lurk in our minds. Anxiety and depression, once formidable foes, yield to the balanced chemistry that exercise cultivates. Neurotransmitter levels find equilibrium, conferring a tranquil serenity upon our inner world.

The pursuit of physical fitness, then, becomes a pilgrimage of the body and soul, a sonata of achievement, resilience, and inner peace. In this odyssey, the union of body and mind unfolds, painting a portrait of wellness that transcends the physical realm, for it is in our movements that we discover the profound masterpiece of self.

In the serene practice of disciplines like yoga and tai chi, the spotlight falls upon mindfulness and relaxation, an alchemy that casts a soothing tranquiliser upon the tumultuous waters of anxiety and depression. In the embrace of serene movements, the mind finds respite, and the heart's burdens are lightened.

Venturing into the realm of group exercises or team sports, we step onto a stage of camaraderie and connection. These gatherings are vessels of social interaction, where the feeling of belonging is knit, and the spectre of isolation recedes. Amidst shared pursuits, friendships blossom, and the tendrils of support networks expand. These collective endeavours offer the gift of companionship, where bonds are nurtured, and communities are forged.

Positive exchanges and shared moments within these gatherings are the seeds of self-esteem and self-assurance. In the chorus of shared laughter and achievement, the soul finds validation and confidence takes root.

The palette of physical activities extends to self-expression and creativity. In the cadence of dance and the canvas of expressive movement, emotions flow freely. Here, the spirit finds release, and the psyche finds renewal. In the intricacies of these activities, the threads of mindfulness, camaraderie, and self-expression intertwine, crafting a masterpiece of emotional and psychological harmony. In each step, each breath, and each dance, we find the symphony of our existence, where the pursuit of well-being unfolds as a shared, creative, and deeply mindful journey.

But the magic of exercise extends even further. It becomes the architect of immune strength, summoning the body's defenders to identify and vanquish potentially cancerous cells. In the quietude of our workouts, the immune system awakens, its vigilance sharpened by the pulse of regular exercise.

In the fabric of health, physical activity develops its vibrant threads, each one a testament to the profound impact it has on our well-being. It is a journey of choices, where the path to diabetes prevention and cancer risk reduction is paved with the pace of our steps, the balance of our hormones, and the resilience of our immune system, a cascade of health harmonised by motion.

Regular aerobic exercise breathes life into the lungs, a transformative force for those grappling with respiratory challenges like COPD and asthma. With each inhale and exhale, the lungs expand in capacity and efficiency, granting the gift of easier breathing, a precious reprieve from the confines of breathlessness.

But the magic of exercise extends its reach beyond the respiratory system. It intertwines with the very fabric of cardiovascular health, alleviating the burdens placed upon the heart and lungs. Through targeted exercises, we empower the very engines of our respiration, forging a path toward improved lung function and heightened respiratory efficiency.

As we shed excess weight, the burden upon our respiratory systems lightens. Breathing becomes less onerous, the path to respite more attainable, and the perils of respiratory conditions are held at bay. In the beat of motion, we uncover not only the means to prevent obesity but the keys to liberation from the shackles of compromised breathing.

Each step we take, each inhale we savour, carries us further along the journey of well-being, a tapestry woven with threads crafted through the intertwining of resilience, vitality, and the triumph of the indomitable human spirit.

Moderate-intensity exercises serves as a catalyst, momentarily boosting the presence of immune cells, particularly those entrusted with immune surveillance. These vigilant cells traverse the body's terrain, diligently scouting for potential adversaries. In post-exercise, there typically ensues a brief surge in the circulation of these immune soldiers, a flow that gradually abates as the body resumes its resting state.

Exercise operates as a regulatory mechanism to produce cytokines, those complex signalling molecules that wield considerable influence over the domain of inflammation. This meticulous orchestration of cytokine production contributes to a harmonious equilibrium, diminishing the susceptibility to chronic, low-grade inflammation.

Moreover, physical activity lends its support to the impeccable functioning of an array of immune warriors. Among them, Natural Killer (NK) cells stand as vigilant patrols, with the capacity to eliminate both virus-infected and cancerous cells.

At this juncture, the virtue of regular exercise becomes evident, as it ignites the activity of these NK cells, thereby elevating the level of immune surveillance. Further reinforcing the body's immune arsenal are the macrophages, voracious cells dedicated to engulfing and annihilating pathogens and cellular debris. In this regard, exercise shines as a promoter of efficiency and responsiveness, bolstering the capabilities of these essential cellular defenders.

The insidious grip of chronic stress has been shown to exact a toll on the immune system, rendering it more vulnerable. In this challenging landscape, physical activity emerges as a formidable antidote, countering stress and its detrimental effects on immune function. One of exercise's pivotal roles lies in its ability to orchestrate the regulation of cortisol, the stress hormone itself.

Elevated cortisol levels have the disquieting power to suppress immune function, making the act of cortisol management through exercise a wise endeavour. Furthermore, physical activity bestows upon us the gift of heightened blood circulation, a phenomenon that aids in the efficient transportation of immune cells and antibodies to every nook and cranny of the body. This swift mobilisation equips immune cells to promptly reach areas marked by infection or inflammation, acting as our body's first responders.

The complex lymphatic system, a foundation of our immune response, is also stirred into action by regular physical activity. Exercise stimulates the flow of lymph which is the silent carrier of immune cells and the eliminator of waste products from our tissues. Exercise lends unwavering support to immune function. Beyond cortisol regulation and lymphatic flow, there exists another facet of immunity intertwined with physical activity, the realm of gut health.

Our gut microbiota, the flourishing community of microorganisms within us, wields a profound influence on immune function. Here, regular physical activity becomes the focal point, nurturing a balanced microbiome and refining our immune responses, creating yet another layer of defence in our arsenal against illness.

The virtue of routine exercise unveils its considerable influence particularly in the sphere of slumber. For, it is beneath the shroud of night that our immune system rejuvenates and fortifies its defences. Scientific understanding reveals that sound sleep is the cornerstone upon which a resilient immune edifice is erected. Slumber begets a crescendo of immune cell production and restoration, it is during these hallowed hours that our body's defenders are diligently sculpted, and their battle scars meticulously healed.

With unwavering commitment to physical activity, our biological orchestra attunes itself to the melody of resilience. The stage upon which this drama unfolds witnesses an uptick in immune cell creation, a refining of their efficacy, and an expeditious reply to foreign invasions. In the theatre of inoculation, exercise takes the lead role, spotlighting its ability to enhance our body's response to vaccinations.

Like an artisan refining a masterpiece, exercise amplifies the creation of antibodies in reaction to vaccine antigens. This mechanism culminates in a robust bastion of immunity. Thus, it should be known that regular exercise, the tireless conductor of this life, bestows upon us not only the gift of restful sleep but also the armour of fortified immunity.

Participating in consistent physical activity bestows upon our bodies a wealth of health benefits. Among its notable virtues lies its prowess in curbing the accumulation of adipose tissue, with a particular emphasis on the pernicious visceral fat, stealthily ensconced around our vital organs. Visceral fat, infamous for its penchant for releasing pro-inflammatory agents, succumbs to the persuasive influence of exercise, diminishing its production and thereby alleviating the scourge of inflammation.

The transformative effects of exercise do not cease at the adipose layer. Rather, they venture deeper, penetrating the inner temple of our cells, where the mighty mitochondria reign supreme as the architects of energy production.

Exercise orchestrates profound adaptations within these cellular dynamos, nurturing their functionality and reducing the generation of malevolent free radicals during the alchemical process of energy creation. These benevolent adjustments, in turn, foster a state of enhanced cellular well-being, where the dividends of exercise are reaped at the most fundamental level of our existence.

Routine physical activity triggers the intricate machinery of DNA repair hidden within our cells. In this remarkable process, our genetic blueprint receives a protective shield against the corrosive effects of oxidative stress, thereby diminishing the peril of cellular malfunction and genetic mutations. In more straightforward terms, exercise emerges as a pivotal proponent in nurturing a healthier physique. It achieves this by mitigating inflammation, enhancing cellular vitality, and serving as a guardian of our genetic heritage.

Exercise orchestrates a ballet of metabolic prowess, enabling muscle cells to welcome glucose with open arms, sans the beckoning call of insulin. This phenomenon holds particular significance for those grappling with insulin resistance, offering a glimmer of hope in the realm of metabolic health. Yet, the virtuosity of physical activity extends beyond the cellular realm, reaching into the delicate balance of hunger and satiety.

It wields an influence over the hormonal duet of leptin and ghrelin, the maestros of appetite regulation. Here, exercise strikes a harmonious chord by lowering the crescendo of ghrelin, the notorious hunger hormone, while fine-tuning the sensitivity of leptin. This ultimately conducts a chorus of improved appetite control.

Consistent exercise wields a profound influence on thyroid function, orchestrating an intricate interplay of hormones that elevate metabolic expertise. Within this process, the conversion of thyroid hormones is refined, contributing to an overall boost in metabolism. A star player in this metabolic mechanism is adiponectin, a hormone crafted by our fat cells.

Adiponectin takes centre stage, bolstering the work of metabolic well-being. It achieves this feat by enhancing the sensitivity of our cells to insulin, ushering in a state of improved responsiveness. In tandem, it unfurls its anti-inflammatory banner, quelling the fires of inflammation that can disrupt metabolic harmony.

As we engage in physical exertion, the body responds with a surge of norepinephrine and epinephrine, commonly known as adrenaline. These hormonal messengers fan the flames of alertness, infusing us with a potent dose of energy and sharpening our focus.

In this grand performance, exercise does not merely stop at invigorating the internal mechanisms of our physiology, it also ushers in a phenomenon known as exercise-induced thermogenesis. At this point, the body generates heat, akin to a furnace stoking its fires. This process is a contributing force behind heightened energy expenditure and an elevated metabolic tempo, propelling us toward greater vitality.

The pursuit of safe and efficacious exercise among our older generation demands meticulous forethought, a deliberate arrangement that considers the nuanced tapestry of their physiological, health, and mobility requisites. In the area of fitness, a well-crafted physical regimen holds the promise of bestowing a treasure trove of advantages, heightened strength, restored equilibrium, fortified cardiovascular resilience, and an overall enhancement of well-being.

Yet, this journey is not embarked upon lightly. It necessitates a judicious weighing of critical factors to ensure that each stride taken is both secure and fruitful. Foremost, prior to the inception of any exercise program, the sage counsel of a healthcare provider should be diligently sought. This counsel is particularly paramount for those harbouring pre-existing medical conditions or those tangled with a web of medications.

A medical evaluation unfurls its cloak, pinpointing any contraindications or precautions that must be adhered to during specific exercises. It serves as the guardian of well-being, guiding our senior population toward a path of vitality and longevity, where each step is trodden with care, wisdom, and a keen eye for individual needs.

The crafting of exercise programs is an art that demands meticulous attention to the unique collage of everyone's fitness level, prevailing health status, and aspirations. Within this opus, we must weave in considerations for existing health conditions, the suppleness of joints, the vigour of muscles, and the delicate equilibrium of balance.

For our cherished older adults, the spectre of falls looms as a significant concern. To counter this peril, exercise programs must develop a combination of activities that serve as sentinels, guardians of balance and coordination. These exercises stand as bastions, diligently working to reduce the precipice of falls and their consequences.

Yet, in this process of movement, we must not overlook the virtues of suppleness. Regular forays of stretching and flexibility exercises emerge as our allies, preserving the mobility of joints and the vast range of motion they bestow. It is through gentle stretching routines that we ward off the unwelcome guest of stiffness, ensuring that the body remains a temple of fluidity and grace.

Commence with the gentlest of exercises, an introduction marked by low-intensity rhythms, and with time, let the tempo ascend in a measured cadence. This deliberate ascent, like a careful climber scaling a peak, permits the body to adjust, ensuring safety in every stride.

For our treasured older adults, the compass of thirst perception may wane with age, making it imperative to sound the clarion call of hydration, a chorus that begins before the overture, dances through the performance, and lingers beyond the final bow. In this masterpiece, each drop of water plays its part in warding off the desiccation that lurks in the wings.

The overture, a gentle prelude, heralds the coming act. A warm-up, it's called, a tender invitation to the body's orchestra to tune its instruments. Blood flows in a rising crescendo, muscles stretch their limbs, preparing for the grand performance. And as the final curtain draws near, do not hasten to exit the stage. Allow for a gentle coda, a cool-down, a denouement to the opus.

The heart, with grace, eases its tempo, the muscles yield with pliancy, a serenade to prevent the stiffness that lingers in the shadows. Listen to the body's whispers, for exercise should not summon pain. If pain, like an unwelcome guest, makes an appearance, let the curtain fall. Seek the counsel of a healthcare sage to unveil the underlying mysteries and pave the way for a harmonious encore.

The choice of footwear cannot be understated, for it becomes the steadfast companion in the journey of physical exertion, offering the solace of support and the embrace of cushioning. Especially in weight-bearing exercises, these allies stand as guards against the presence of injury. Between the beats of exercise, pause to allow time for restoration. These interludes are not mere respites but vital intermissions that safeguard against the perils of overuse, nurturing the body's innate healing mechanisms.

Engage in the camaraderie of group exercise, where shared effort fosters not only social connections but also the ember of motivation. With each endeavour, the older soul must embark as both traveller and cartographer. A vigilant monitor of progress, noting the subtle shifts in fitness, mobility, and the overarching arras of well-being.

Yet, in this odyssey of movement, the compass of enjoyment must not be neglected. The terrain of exercise should be diverse, the activities engaging, for it is in the embrace of enjoyment that motivation takes root and commitment to the regimen remains unwavering.

In the composition of effective and secure physical activity, the tailor's art finds its place, crafting bespoke exercise programs that seamlessly align with unique individual needs and capabilities. The human being, a masterpiece of diversity, bears no replica. Herein, factors as diverse as the strands of fitness, health, age, medical intricacies, and personal aspirations converge to chart the course of a distinct exercise odyssey.

Within this tailor-made narrative lies a steadfast commitment to safety, for the bespoke garment of exercise considers every nuance, each medical thread, every injury's impact, and every limitation's hue. Here, individualised exercise programs emerge as the vigilant guardians of well-being, ensuring that each movement aligns harmoniously with one's unique circumstances.

In contrast, the pre-made, one-size-fits-all garb, while convenient, may inadvertently unravel the fabric of safety. It risks misalignment with individual intricacies, elevating the presence of injuries, exacerbating health complexities, or pushing the boundaries of endurance to the brink.

The harmonious alignment of exercises with an individual's unique needs and capacities paves a path toward the bespoke acquisition of health benefits. It is a journey tailored to the very essence of one's well-being, where precision reigns supreme. Consider, for instance, the individual with osteoporosis, for whom exercises akin to a guardian's embrace are tailored to nurture bone health. Likewise, another soul, facing the shadow of cardiovascular risk, finds solace in aerobic pursuits that fan the flames of heart health.

In this bespoke endeavour, the compass of goals is finely calibrated to the individual's present fitness coordinates and life's circumstances. It is a symphony in which the notes of achievement are not merely penned but sung aloud. Motivation, then, thrives as progress unfurls its banner, and the fruits of labour materialise in full view, tangible evidence of unwavering dedication.

The fibre that twists commitment into the fabric of an exercise routine is the alignment of one's passions, capabilities, and aspirations. A sonata composed to cater to individual interests and goals not only inspires dedication but also nurtures the enduring embrace of physical activity.

Within this bespoke tapestry lies the secret of adherence, an unwavering commitment that defies the whims of time. Custom-tailored programs, like a skilled conductor, fine-tunes the rhythm to each individual's unique composition. They gracefully navigate around the physical boundaries and medical nuances, ensuring that exercise remains a haven for all.

Consider, for instance, the individual with knee afflictions, who finds succour in the gentle pace of low-impact activities, a comfort to ease joint strain. Likewise, someone grappling with diabetes would benefit from exercises that harmonise with blood sugar regulation.

But the beauty of a tailored program is its adaptability. It evolves with the climax of one's fitness journey, adjusting to higher notes as the body grows stronger. In this gradual progression, the exercises remain a stimulating challenge, bequeathing benefits without ever courting the risk of injury or burnout.

Tailored fitness programs, thoughtfully crafted to align with one's unique preferences and passions, hold the potential to accelerate a philosophical transformation in one's overall well-being. Such personalised regimens unveil an array of benefits, harmoniously resonating through the corridors of mental fortitude, motivation, and an unswerving contentment with the exercise journey. In this finely tuned approach to fitness, the invaluable charm lies in its ability to gracefully sidestep the dreaded plateaus that often hinder progress.

By perpetually refreshing and recalibrating exercise programs, individuals are offered an unending propel of improvement, a continuous ascension in strength, endurance, flexibility, and other vital components of physical fitness.

Yet, the true artistry of personalised programs resides in their unwavering focus on exercises that are intrinsically attuned to the individual's goals. In this way, they serve as vigilant guardians against the inefficacy of time spent on activities that do not harmonise with the noble pursuits etched within the individual's aspirations.

Triumphing in exercises that align seamlessly with one's unique abilities nurtures the seeds of self-assurance and self-worth. This affirmative feedback loop constructs a weighty sense of achievement, serving as a beckoning beacon for ongoing engagement. In the artful instrumentation of one's fitness journey, collaboration with a seasoned fitness professional or a knowledgeable healthcare provider takes centre stage. It establishes a sturdy scaffold of support and leverages their expertise as a compass, diligently steering individuals towards the shores of their aspirations.

The tapestry of longevity and holistic well-being is intricately woven from the threads of physical activity, dietary choices, and quality of sleep. These facets of life, in their corresponding interplay, conspire to extend one's health span and ultimately, one's lifespan.

At the nexus of this sophisticated interplay, physical activity takes centre stage. It is the fulcrum in the maintenance of a finely tuned energy equilibrium. When partnered with a well-balanced diet, its role becomes pivotal in averting the perils of excessive weight gain or loss, a hazardous tightrope walk that is closely entwined with the onset of numerous chronic maladies and the subtle, yet profound, ripples they cast upon the canvas of longevity.

The tempo of consistent physical activity coordinates a symphony of metabolic enhancements, coaxing forth the body's innate capacity to wield nutrients with precision and grace. In this delicate interplay, digestion finds its cadence, nutrient absorption its resonance, and metabolic health its harmonious pulse.

Exercise, as both maestro and muse, wields its influence over the subtle mechanisms governing our appetite. It conducts a subtle concerto with hormones like leptin and ghrelin, composing them to ward off the siren song of overindulgence, and thus, treads the path of weight management with finesse.

The temporal interplay between meals and exercise yields profound effects on our vitality, the upsurge of our workout performances, and the tender, post-exertion process of recovery.

In this finely tuned process, well-timed nutrition takes on the role of the instrumentalist, delivering the essential nutrients that form the cornerstone of peak exercise performance and the subsequent renewal of the body.

This interplay extends to the realm of sleep, where the intelligence of regular physical activity unfolds. By kindling the fires of restorative rest, it gifts us with deeper, more profound sleep. However, the chronology of our exertions carries weight. The fervour of strenuous activity too close to bedtime can cast a shadow on the realm of dreams, potentially impinging upon our delicate repose.

Conversely, when the day's light finds us engaged in daytime physical pursuits, it serves as the maestro, conducting the delicate work of circadian rhythms, ultimately bestowing upon us the gift of enhanced sleep duration and quality.

Physical activity is a well-documented antidote to the burdens of stress and anxiety, its soothing embrace promoting a tranquil state of mind conducive to restful slumber. It gracefully casts aside the tumultuous thoughts that often besiege us in the nocturnal hours, paving the way for uninterrupted sleep. The role of diet in this nocturnal ballet is equally noteworthy. Certain foods, graced with nutrients like magnesium and tryptophan, assume the role of soporific virtuosos, serenading us into states of relaxation and deeper sleep.

Yet, sleep is also sensitive to the discordant notes of caffeine and sugar, particularly when consumed in the evening. Their restrained consumption serves as a guardian against sleep disturbances and the capricious fluctuations in blood sugar levels. In this nocturnal journey, hydration is a faithful companion. Maintaining adequate fluid levels throughout the day ensures a hydrated fabric upon which the drapery of sleep can be artfully woven, preventing the jarring awakenings that thirst may summon in the quiet of night.

In the intricate complexities of well-being, the triumvirate of physical activity, a well-balanced diet, and restorative sleep emerges as the guardians of vitality. Together, they wield their collective influence to quell the fiery tempest of chronic inflammation, a formidable instigator of ageing and its associated maladies.

Their appropriate alliance extends its protective mantle to the domain of cardiovascular health, deftly lowering the spectre of heart disease, stroke, and other vascular adversaries. By nurturing stable blood sugar levels, preserving insulin sensitivity, and maintaining a harmonious body weight, this cooperation of lifestyle choices forms an impervious shield against the encroachments of type 2 diabetes and metabolic syndrome.

However, their beneficence doesn't cease at the borders of the body, it permeates the recesses of the mind. These lifestyle factors are instrumental in safeguarding cognitive prowess and the sanctuary of brain health, repelling the shadows of neurodegenerative ailments like dementia.

In their splendid interplay, physical activity, diet, and sleep don the mantles of wellness architects, crafting a life of unparalleled physical, mental, and emotional harmony. Through their diligent ministrations, they bestow upon us the gift of enriched existence and the promise of an enduring journey toward longevity.

Chapter 6 – Rest and Recovery: The importance of Sleep and Stress Management

Rest and recovery, those quintessential pillars of holistic well-being, constitute the exquisite mechanisms through which both body and mind experience restoration, rejuvenation, and revival following the trials of life. Physical rest, the art of allowing the corporeal vessel to gently surrender to serenity, assumes the mantle of respite from the ceaseless demands of activity and exertion.

During this interlude of tranquillity, the body meticulously hoards its precious energy, elegantly lowering the heart's metronome, and gracefully unwinding every taut muscle fibre. Such restful symphony can manifest as slumber, a serene reprieve, or the mindful reduction of physical strain. In this harmonious pause, the body embraces the delicate choreography of healing and renewal, dancing with grace to the cadence of its own restoration.

In the delicate realm of the mind, mental rest emerges as an art of quietude, an intermission from the ceaseless flurry of cognitive activity and the weight of mental toil. Here, we tread upon the grounds of serenity, embarking on the winding paths of meditation, mindfulness, or the enchanting pursuits that grant the intellect a soothing refuge. Mental rest unfurls as a reverie, where the mind is set free to wander, unfettered and unburdened. In this tranquil sanctuary, the fruits of focus, creativity, and cognitive prowess ripen and thrive.

Emotional rest, a sanctuary for the heart's tumultuous tides, stands as the sentinel against the emotional tempests that seek to weary the soul. It is the craft of taming and appeasing the emotional torrents, akin to a gentle conductor orchestrating a symphony of well-being.

Here, one finds solace in the catharsis of emotional expression, in the profound dialogues with compassionate counsellors and therapists, and in the tender embrace of activities that wrap the heart in comfort. Emotional rest, the guardian of emotional equilibrium, weaves a resolute defence against the spectre of burnout and stands as the sanctuary of emotional prosperity.

In the sphere of well-being, physical recovery emerges as the body's convalescence and adaptation in the wake of strenuous exertion. At this time, we embrace the nurturing of elements such as the balm of adequate sleep, the sustenance of wholesome nutrition, the elixir of hydration, and the harmonious cadence of activities dedicated to the revitalisation and mending of our tireless muscles.

In this sanctuary of rejuvenation, physical recovery unfurls as the nurturing gardener, tending to the blooms of strength, the blossoms of endurance, and the masterpiece of overall physical prowess.

Mental recovery, the cherished refuge for our cerebral sanctum, stands as the guardian of mental vitality and resilience. It is the sanctuary where the mind, an ethereal vessel, finds its well-deserved reprieve. Here, we commune with the enchanting rituals of relaxation, traverse the ethereal realms of mindfulness, and embark on soul-enriching forays into the realms of recreation.

In this orbit of serenity, mental fatigue dissolves like morning mist, anxiety retreats like shadows at dawn, and mental clarity and decision-making flourish like a garden in full bloom. In the tapestry of holistic well-being, the harmonious dance of physical and mental recovery takes centre stage, a ballet of rejuvenation that nourishes both body and soul.

In the tender embrace of well-being's collage, emotional recovery emerges as the diligent caretaker of our heart's serenity and resilience. It is the concerto of self-compassion, the dance of shared burdens, and the refuge of activities that breathe life into our emotional sanctuary. Here, we embark on the pilgrimage of nurturing our emotional garden, allowing it to bloom in full splendour.

Emotional recovery, the guardian of the heart's equilibrium, extends its nurturing hand to guide us through the labyrinth of stress, shielding us from the spectre of emotional exhaustion, and bestowing upon us the cherished gift of emotional equilibrium.

Rest and recovery rise as the architects of our corporeal well-being, they are the masterminds behind the mending of muscles and tissues, the artisans of strength, and the custodians of the immune sentinels. Adequate rest, a resplendent comfort, whispers to the body, bidding it to repair and strengthen, to rejuvenate and renew.

In its absence, physical fatigue casts its shadows, injuries loom like silent glooms, and the immune fortress stands vulnerable. The gentle ministrations of rest and recovery sculpt the pillars of physical vigour, an essential foundation in the palace of health.

Amidst the intricacies of the human consciousness, the gentle embrace of mental repose and recovery holds the power to diminish the weight of mental strain, serving as a bulwark against the encroachment of afflictions such as anxiety and depression.

To unlock this sanctuary of tranquillity, one must unlock the twin gates of quality sleep and the artful techniques of relaxation, for within their depths lies the elixir of mental rejuvenation, the steadfast guardians of cognitive vigour.

In the ethereal realm of emotions, the art of emotional rest and recovery unfurls its benevolent wings, cradling the weary heart and spirit. In its tender care, emotional resilience finds its nurturing sanctuary, burnout is banished, and the tapestry of emotional well-being is woven with delicate threads of hope.

In the intricate dance of life, addressing emotional stress emerges as an imperative task, as it forges the sturdy bonds of healthy relationships and equips us with the tools to navigate the turbulent waters of life's tribulations.

Seasoned athletes and those who pursue the pinnacle of human performance are well-acquainted with the profound importance of rest and recuperation in the quest to refine both physical prowess and mental acumen. The art of proper recovery is the cornerstone upon which enhanced endurance, amplified strength and athletic achievement are woven.

Moreover, the faithful devotion to the rituals of rest and rejuvenation does not merely serve as a fleeting indulgence, it emerges as a weighty investment in the currency of longevity and vitality, mitigating the looming presence of chronic ailments while bestowing the gift of an enriched and fuller existence.

Yet, the science of slumber, that enigmatic voyage into the nocturnal realms of consciousness, beckons with its intricate charm. To delve into the esoteric world of sleep science is to embark on a voyage through the labyrinthine corridors of human physiology.

Herein lie the inscrutable cycles, the beguiling stages, and the orchestrations of circadian rhythms that preside over the nocturnal theatre of our subconscious. To grasp the science behind slumber is to fathom the delicate dance that unfolds each night, one whose rhythms resonate with the cadence of life itself.

Sleep is a nuanced journey rather than a monotonous state, characterised by intricate cycles. Two key phases shape these cycles, Rapid Eye Movement (REM) sleep and Non-Rapid Eye Movement (NREM) sleep. These phases gracefully unfold multiple times throughout a night's rest. The NREM sleep phase encompasses three discernible stages, N1, N2, and N3. N1, also known as Stage 1, serves as the transitional threshold from wakefulness to sleep.

During this phase, muscular activity dwindles, and eye movements adopt a leisurely pace, marking a gentle introduction to the realm of slumber. Progressing to N2, or Stage 2, a cessation of eye movements takes place, accompanied by a synchronisation of brain activity. This stage, characterised by a more profound level of sleep, deepens the voyage into the nocturnal landscape.

Entering N3, recognised as Stage 3 and often referred to as slow-wave sleep, one delves into the profound depths of NREM sleep. Marked by unhurried, high-amplitude brain waves, this stage orchestrates a symphony of crucial bodily functions. It is in the embrace of N3 that processes such as cell repair, growth, and the fortification of the immune system reach their zenith.

On the contrary, REM sleep paints a contrasting tableau with its rapid eye movements, heightened brain activity, and the vibrant tapestry of dreams. This stage holds a pivotal role in cognitive functions, acting as a maestro orchestrating the consolidation of memory and the regulation of emotions. The inaugural REM cycle typically unfolds approximately 90 minutes after the initial descent into slumber, and its duration extends with each subsequent cycle, weaving a dynamic pattern throughout the night.

The arrangement of NREM and REM sleep stages in a night's sleep forms a specific sleep architecture. A typical sleep cycle consists of N1, N2, N3, and REM stages, followed by the next cycle, with each cycle lasting approximately 90 minutes. As the night progresses, the proportion of REM sleep increases, while N3 deep sleep decreases.

Circadian rhythms are internal, biological clocks that regulate various physiological processes, including sleep-wake cycles. The suprachiasmatic nucleus (SCN) in the brain's hypothalamus serves as the body's master clock, receiving light signals from the eyes to synchronise the body's internal clock with the external day-night cycle.

Circadian tempos dictate our natural sleep-wake patterns. The hormone melatonin, produced by the pineal gland, plays a crucial role in sleep regulation. Melatonin levels rise in the evening, signalling the body to prepare for sleep. Disruption of circadian rhythms, such as shift work or jet lag, can lead to sleep disturbances and various health issues. Night-shift workers often struggle with sleep difficulties and are at a higher risk of conditions like obesity, diabetes, and mood disorders.

The repercussions of insufficient sleep, be it chronic or fleeting, cast a profound and deleterious shadow upon diverse facets of an individual's health and well-being. From the corporeal realm to cognitive prowess and emotional equilibrium, the toll exacted by sleep deprivation is far-reaching. This challenge is further compounded by the intricate landscape of sleep disorders.

Persistent deprivation of sleep intertwines with a heightened vulnerability to hypertension, heart disease, and stroke. It disrupts the delicate equilibrium of blood pressure regulation and elevates stress hormone levels, notably cortisol. Moreover, the consequences extend to metabolic pathways, where sleep deprivation disrupts glucose metabolism and undermines insulin sensitivity, escalating the risk of type 2 diabetes and obesity. Notably, it fans the flames of appetite, often steering individuals towards suboptimal dietary choices.

The intricate interplay between sleep and immune system function underscores the pivotal role of rest in safeguarding overall health. Deprivation of sleep, conversely, emerges as a catalyst for compromise, rendering individuals more susceptible to infections. Beyond its immunological significance, sleep assumes a leading role in cognitive vitality and memory consolidation.

Regrettably, the consequences of sleep deprivation manifest in a compromised capacity to absorb new information and retain facts. The repercussions extend to diminished attention span, waning alertness, and compromised decision-making, predisposing individuals to accidents and errors. In the long term, sustained sleep deprivation may contribute to cognitive decline and elevate the risk of neurodegenerative conditions such as Alzheimer's.

Sleep deprivation can lead to mood swings, irritability, and increased emotional reactivity. It is strongly associated with symptoms of anxiety and depression. Lack of sleep can amplify the body's stress response, making it more challenging to cope with stressors and contributing to chronic stress. Adequate sleep is crucial for emotional regulation and resilience.

Sleep-deprived individuals may struggle to manage their emotions effectively. Insomnia is characterised by difficulty falling asleep or staying asleep, leading to insufficient sleep and impaired daytime functioning. It is one of the most common sleep disorders, affecting millions of people worldwide. Both acute and chronic insomnia are prevalent.

Sleep apnea manifests as recurrent disruptions in breathing during sleep, fostering fleeting awakenings and diminishing the overall quality of rest. A considerable segment of the population, particularly those carrying excess weight, is believed to grapple with undiagnosed sleep apnea.

Restless Legs Syndrome (RLS), a neurological affliction, manifests as an irresistible compulsion to move the legs, often accompanied by disconcerting sensations. This condition afflicts a substantial number of individuals, inducing disturbances in sleep and persistent discomfort during waking hours.

Narcolepsy, a rare neurological disorder, is distinguished by an overwhelming daytime drowsiness, abrupt loss of muscle control (cataplexy), and vivid dreaming. Though less prevalent, narcolepsy can wield a significant impact on an individual's daily life.

The perils of sleep deprivation extend across various dimensions, encompassing physical health, cognitive function, and emotional well-being. Grasping the intricacies of these detrimental effects becomes imperative in underscoring the significance of prioritising sleep and acknowledging the importance of identifying and addressing sleep disorders. Championing the cultivation of healthy sleep habits and promptly seeking medical intervention when needed emerges as pivotal measures in alleviating the adverse repercussions of sleep deprivation.

Distinguishing between the quantity and quality of sleep is a pivotal consideration when delving into the significance of sleep for holistic well-being. The crucial role of rest in sustaining both physical and mental health hinges on both the duration and the calibre of one's sleep.

Quantity, denoting the total time allocated to rest, is typically measured in hours. While the recommended amount varies with age, adults generally benefit from 7-9 hours per night. Factors such as age, genetics, and individual requirements contribute to determining the optimal quantity of sleep for an individual.

Conversely, the quality of sleep pertains to the restorative and rejuvenating aspects of one's sleep, transcending mere hours spent in bed. It is defined by the depth and efficacy of your rest. Numerous factors contribute to sleep quality, among which are sleep cycles. A standard sleep cycle comprises distinct stages, encompassing both REM (rapid eye movement) and non-REM phases.

The non-REM stages, characterised by deep and revitalising sleep, contrast with the REM stage, linked to dreaming. Achieving a harmonious transition through these stages proves indispensable for ensuring a high standard of sleep.

Sleep disruptions, characterised by frequent awakenings, disturbances, or conditions like sleep apnea, have the potential to disrupt sleep cycles and diminish overall sleep quality. The sleep environment also plays a pivotal role, with factors such as noise, light, room temperature, and the comfort of your mattress and pillows significantly influencing the quality of sleep. Additionally, sleep disorders such as insomnia, restless leg syndrome, and narcolepsy pose challenges to maintaining optimal sleep quality.

Quality sleep supports improved memory, problem-solving, creativity, and overall cognitive function. It aids in consolidating and organising information. It is essential for regulating mood and emotional stability. It can reduce the risk of mood disorders, such as depression and anxiety.

High-quality sleep is linked to improved cardiovascular health, effective weight management, and a robust immune system. It serves as a mitigating factor against the risk of chronic conditions such as diabetes and hypertension. For athletes, high-quality sleep plays a pivotal role in facilitating recovery, promoting muscle repair, and enhancing overall athletic performance. Consistent access to restful, high-quality sleep is correlated with a longer, healthier lifespan.

Optimal sleep quality serves as a powerful tool for the effective management of stress, diminishing the production of stress hormones and fostering a state of relaxation. This, in turn, translates into heightened focus and increased productivity during waking hours.

Elevating the quality of your sleep involves cultivating good sleep hygiene, crafting a comfortable sleep environment, and addressing any underlying sleep disorders. While both the quantity and quality of sleep are integral to overall well-being, the enhancement of sleep quality holds the potential for profound and far-reaching benefits for both physical and mental health.

Stress emerges as a natural and adaptive reaction to diverse external or internal stimuli, presenting either a threat or challenge to an individual. Within moderate bounds, stress proves motivational, propelling us to effectively confront potential threats. However, the persistence of chronic or excessive stress can induce profound physiological and psychological impacts on the body.

At the heart of the body's response to stress lies the release of stress hormones, with cortisol taking centre stage. Triggered by the brain's perception of a stressor, cortisol is unleashed from the adrenal glands. Operating as a linchpin in the body's stress response, cortisol readies the body for a "fight or flight" reaction, elevating heart rate, intensifying focus, and supplying a surge of energy.

The activation of the sympathetic nervous system by stress initiates a surge in both heart rate and blood pressure. With the passage of time, persistent stress becomes a contributing factor to hypertension, posing a heightened risk for cardiovascular diseases. The enduring impact of stress extends to the immune system, gradually compromising its resilience against infections and illnesses. This vulnerability is attributed to the prolonged exposure to stress hormones such as cortisol, which, in turn, has the capacity to suppress immune function.

The repercussions of stress extend to the digestive system, giving rise to complications like indigestion, acid reflux, and irritable bowel syndrome (IBS). The "fight or flight" response triggered by stress has the potential to redirect blood flow away from the digestive organs.

Concurrently, stress frequently manifests as muscle tension, precipitating or intensifying conditions such as tension headaches and musculoskeletal pain. In addition, stress can disturb sleep patterns, culminating in insomnia or poor-quality sleep. This compounds the already considerable physical and psychological toll of stress.

Persistent stress emerges as a significant precursor to anxiety disorders and depression, with elevated cortisol levels exerting an influence on brain function and exacerbating mood disorders. The cognitive fallout of stress is evident in impaired memory, compromised decision-making, and diminished concentration, particularly prevalent in those grappling with chronic stress.

Emotional repercussions are equally pronounced, as stress can instigate emotional instability, mood oscillations, and heightened irritability. Furthermore, pre-existing emotional conditions may be aggravated by the impact of stress.

Stress often prompts behavioural shifts in individuals, manifesting as alterations in eating habits, substance misuse, and a propensity for increased risk-taking. Extended exposure to stress elevates the likelihood of developing mental health disorders, including post-traumatic stress disorder (PTSD).

Recognising the profound influence of stress on both physiological and psychological facets is paramount for effective management and mitigation of its effects. Implementing stress management strategies such as mindfulness, relaxation techniques, exercise, and seeking guidance from healthcare professionals or therapists, becomes crucial for preserving both physical and mental well-being amidst the challenges posed by stress.

The intricate interplay between stress, sleep, and overall health stands as a pivotal facet in comprehending human well-being. Stress and sleep share a bidirectional relationship, exerting mutual influence and affecting diverse aspects of physical and mental health.

Delving into stress and its repercussions on sleep, we find that stress can disturb sleep patterns, causing challenges in falling asleep, maintaining sleep, or attaining restorative rest. Those under stress often contend with racing thoughts, elevated heart rate, and heightened alertness, factors that impede their capacity to unwind and achieve a restful night's sleep.

Extended periods of stress can intricately weave a troublesome narrative with insomnia, a condition marked by the intricate struggles of finding solace in the embrace of sleep. Chronic stress, the relentless storyteller, tells a tale of heightened arousal, disrupting the delicate ebb and flow of our natural sleep-wake cycle. In this narrative, stress becomes the maestro orchestrating nightmares and night sweats, casting a shadow that prompts frequent awakenings in the stillness of the night, stealing away the chance for deep, restorative slumber.

This enduring stress, this persistent plotline, becomes entangled with the threads of sleep disorders, spinning a complex tapestry of unrest. It beckons forth sleep apnea, restless leg syndrome, and the dissonance of circadian rhythm disorders, each playing a distinct role in this nocturnal drama.

The consequence of this prolonged stress is an intricate dance between the waking world and the realm of dreams, leaving the weary protagonist yearning for the elusive tranquillity that restful sleep promises. In this narrative of chronic stress, the risk of sleep disorders stands as a poignant subplot, a reminder that the consequences of a tumultuous mind extend beyond the waking hours, seeping into the sanctuary of the night.

Where stress holds its sway, the delicate embroidery of sleep undergoes a subtle but profound transformation. As stress levels ascend, the serenity of sleep descends, carving a narrative where the two are in a tandem of turmoil. The complex interplay unfolds as poor sleep quality intertwines with heightened stress, each feeding into the other with a relentless rhythm, creating a cycle of unrest. In this choreography of stress, cortisol emerges as the hero, a stress hormone that, when unleashed, disrupts the body's natural cadence.

Circadian rhythms falter, and the harmonious sleep-wake cycle falters under its influence. The consequence is a dissonance that echoes in the quiet hours of the night, impairing the sanctuary of rest. This symbiotic relationship between stress and sleep extends its tendrils into the vast landscape of mental health.

Chronic stress, the maestro of discord, conducts the development of anxiety and depression, shadows that often dance in tandem with sleep disturbances. Conversely, the insufficiency or inadequate quality of sleep assumes its role as a silent contributor to the emergence of mood disorders, completing the intricate and nuanced interplay between the realms of stress, sleep, and mental well-being.

Slumber stands as an indispensable ally, fostering the body's intricate recovery and self-restoration. When stress barges in, disrupting the delicate balance of repose, it unfurls a tapestry of potential physical maladies. The immune system falters, the heart contends with unforeseen challenges, and metabolic equilibrium teeters on the edge. Yet, in this symphony of well-being, a remedy lies in the art of stress management.

To fortify the bastion of sound sleep, a strategic approach to stress becomes imperative. Embracing mindfulness, delving into the serenity of meditation, engaging in the rhythmic cadence of deep breathing exercises, and partaking in regular physical activity emerge as the artisans shaping a sanctuary against stress. Through these endeavours, stress levels wane, paving the way for a rejuvenated and more profound slumber, wherein the body reclaims its rightful hours of restoration.

Cultivating a repertoire of sound sleep practices stands pivotal in enhancing the quality of rest. This involves the adherence to a consistent sleep schedule, crafting a tranquil sleep environment, and avoiding stimulants like caffeine and electronic devices in the moments leading up to bedtime.

Delving into the realm of Cognitive-Behavioural Therapy for Insomnia (CBT-I) proves to be an evidence-based approach. This therapeutic modality assists individuals in discerning and tackling the intricacies that contribute to their sleep disruptions, notably stress. Through these thoughtful interventions, the path to improved sleep quality unfolds, fostering a sanctuary for restorative repose.

In certain instances, individuals grappling with profound sleep disruptions or underlying medical conditions may require medical or pharmacological interventions. Recognising the intricate interplay between stress, sleep, and holistic health emphasises the need for a comprehensive approach to well-being.

The crux lies in adeptly navigating the realms of stress management and the cultivation of healthy sleep habits. These measures prove indispensable in upholding both physical and mental health, contributing to the cultivation of a harmonious mind-body connection.

Perennial stress, characterised by the enduring and prolonged exposure to stressors, can exert profound and adverse impacts on both the physical and mental well-being of an individual. While the body's stress response demonstrates adaptability in the short run, its perpetual activation unfolds into a cascade of harm.

Prolonged exposure to chronic stress becomes a harbinger of heightened blood pressure, a pivotal risk factor for heart disease and stroke. The incessant triggering of the stress response manifests in an elevated heart rate and the constriction of blood vessels, culminating in an undesirable surge in blood pressure.

The persistent presence of stress may play a role in fostering the development of atherosclerosis, a condition marked by the accumulation of plaque within the arteries. This insidious process compromises blood flow, heightening the vulnerability to heart attacks and strokes. Notably, stress is a catalyst for arrhythmias, instigating irregular heartbeats, a perilous prospect, particularly for those with pre-existing cardiac conditions.

Furthermore, the ramifications of chronic stress extend to the immune system, where its continuous strain weakens the body's defences against infections and illnesses. Stress hormones, notably cortisol, assume a suppressive role, diminishing the immune response and undermining the body's capacity to ward off pathogens.

For those ensnared by chronic stress, the toll extends beyond the mental realm, permeating the body's defences. Immunity wanes, rendering individuals more susceptible to recurrent colds and infections, while concurrently intensifying the challenges faced by those grappling with pre-existing autoimmune disorders. The repercussions of chronic stress are not confined solely to physical health, they cast a shadow on the delicate balance of mental well-being.

Within the crucible of prolonged stress lies a significant catalyst for anxiety disorders, including but not limited to generalised anxiety disorder and panic disorder. The insidious influence of chronic stress spawns a breeding ground for persistent and disproportionate worry, fostering an atmosphere thick with fear.

The protracted dance with stress is also an architect of melancholy, as it lays the groundwork for the onset of depression. Elevated cortisol levels and subtle shifts in brain chemistry conspire to disrupt mood regulation, ushering in feelings of profound sadness and hopelessness.

When faced with traumatic stressors, particularly when endured chronically, the intricate tapestry of mental health can be tortuously rewoven, resulting in the emergence of Post-Traumatic Stress Disorder (PTSD). This formidable condition unfurls its impact through intrusive thoughts, haunting flashbacks, and a spectrum of emotional distress, underscoring the enduring consequences of trauma.

Turning attention to the corporeal repercussions of chronic stress reveals its insidious link to gastrointestinal maladies. The repertoire of afflictions includes irritable bowel syndrome (IBS), indigestion, and acid reflux, conditions that often bear witness to heightened exacerbation under the weight of stress.

The far-reaching arm of stress extends to the gut microbiome, a vital orchestrator in the opus of digestion and holistic well-being. As stress casts its shadow over this delicate ecosystem, its repercussions ripple through digestive processes and overall health.

The intricate connection between stress and metabolism can give rise to subtle yet profound changes in one's appetite and weight. For some, stress becomes a catalyst for overindulgence, resulting in an unwelcome increase in weight. Conversely, others may find themselves grappling with a loss of appetite, culminating in a noticeable shedding of pounds.

The prolonged embrace of chronic stress can usher in the menacing spectre of insulin resistance, a harbinger of the development of type 2 diabetes. This enduring stress not only disrupts the tranquillity of our waking hours but extends its disruptive tendrils into the realm of sleep, fostering conditions such as insomnia.

Anxiety and incessant thoughts, born from the clutches of stress, conspire to thwart the calm necessary for a restful night. The consequence is a slumber of inferior quality, marked by its elusive nature. Stress, in its relentless pursuit, can manifest physically, weaving itself into the very fabric of our muscles. Tension and pain become unwelcome companions, offering a breeding ground for afflictions like tension headaches and musculoskeletal disorders.

Chronic stress doesn't merely limit its impact to the corporeal realm, it extends its dominion to the realm of enduring pain. Conditions such as fibromyalgia find fertile ground in those who bear the weight of perpetual stress. Thus, the body, in its eloquent response to the trials of life, whispers the toll of stress through the language of discomfort and imbalance.

Delving into the health implications of enduring stress underscores the critical significance of cultivating effective stress management and self-care practices. Navigating the complexities of stress necessitates a repertoire of strategies, encompassing relaxation techniques, mindfulness, physical exercise, the embrace of social support, and, when needed, the therapeutic guidance of counselling or therapy. Consciously acknowledging and proactively addressing chronic stress serves as a proactive measure, working to diminish its adverse effects on both physical health and overall well-being.

Sleep hygiene encompasses a series of mindful practices and habits designed to enhance the quality of sleep and establish a steady sleep pattern. Adhering to these guidelines can aid in cultivating an environment conducive to sleep and refining overall sleep routine. Maintain a consistent bedtime and waking schedule, adhering to it diligently even during weekends. This steadfast routine contributes to the regulation of the body's internal clock.

Introduce soothing pre-sleep rituals, whether it involves reading, enjoying a warm bath, or engaging in relaxation techniques. Steer clear of stimulating activities, such as watching intense TV shows or participating in heated discussions, in the moments leading up to bedtime, this will help foster a tranquil transition into restful sleep.

Craft a serene ambiance in your bedroom by maintaining a cool, quiet, and dark environment. Employ blackout curtains and earplugs to shield yourself from intrusive light and noise. Prioritise your sleep sanctuary with a quality mattress and supportive pillows to ensure optimal comfort.

Diminish screen time, especially exposure to the sleep-disruptive blue light emitted by smartphones, tablets, and computers, at least an hour before bedtime. This precautionary measure mitigates the interference of blue light with melatonin production, the pivotal sleep-regulating hormone.

Steer clear of stimulants like caffeine and nicotine in the hours preceding bedtime, recognising their potential to disrupt your sleep. Sidestep heavy, spicy, and substantial meals close to bedtime to evade discomfort and indigestion, opting for a light snack if hunger persists.

While regular physical activity enhances sleep quality, strive to conclude your workout at least a few hours before bedtime, affording your body the time to ease into a state of rest. Incorporate relaxation techniques like deep breathing, meditation, or progressive muscle relaxation into your pre-sleep routine to alleviate stress and anxiety that could otherwise hinder your ability to unwind.

For daytime naps, opt for brief durations, around 20-30 minutes, and schedule them earlier in the day to prevent any interference with night-time sleep. Abandon the habit of constantly checking the clock, as it can breed anxiety about sleeplessness, exacerbating the challenge of falling asleep. Consider turning the clock away from your line of sight to ease this pressure. Maintain a clear boundary between work, TV, or phone use and your bed. Designate your bed solely for sleep and intimate activities, reinforcing the connection between your bed and rest.

If persistent sleep difficulties, chronic insomnia, or a suspected sleep disorder troubles you, seek guidance and potential treatment from a healthcare professional or a specialised sleep expert. To curtail night-time bathroom visits, limit fluid intake an hour or two before bedtime.

Integrate these sleep hygiene practices into your daily routine to craft an environment conducive to peaceful sleep and cultivate a consistent sleep pattern that fosters overall well-being. Explore these suggestions to discover the optimal combination tailored to your unique sleep requirements.

Sleep disorders wield a substantial influence on an individual's holistic well-being and the quality of their life. Within the realm of common sleep disorders, one encounters the challenges presented by insomnia, sleep apnea, and restless leg syndrome, each characterised by a distinct array of symptoms, diagnostic approaches, and available treatment modalities.

The manifestations of these disorders may include difficulty initiating sleep, recurrent awakenings throughout the night, early morning awakenings coupled with an inability to resume sleep, and non-restorative sleep, leaving one feeling unrefreshed upon waking. These nocturnal disturbances often cast their shadows into the daylight hours, manifesting as daytime fatigue, heightened irritability, and impaired concentration.

The diagnostic process for sleep disorders typically entails a comprehensive assessment conducted by a healthcare provider. Employing a sleep diary to meticulously record sleep patterns and habits is a common practice. In certain instances, a sleep study, known as polysomnography, may be advised to eliminate the possibility of other underlying sleep disorders. Addressing sleep-related concerns often involves a multifaceted approach.

Lifestyle modifications, such as enhancing sleep hygiene through the maintenance of a regular sleep schedule and abstaining from caffeine and alcohol before bedtime, are pivotal. Cognitive-behavioural therapy for insomnia (CBT-I) emerges as an effective intervention, aiming to reshape behaviours and thought patterns contributing to insomnia. In select cases, medications such as sedatives or hypnotics may be prescribed to facilitate improved sleep.

Sleep apnea manifests through distinctive symptoms, encompassing loud and continual snoring, intermittent pauses in breathing during sleep, frequently succeeded by abrupt gasping or choking. Individuals affected often experience excessive daytime sleepiness, morning headaches, challenges in concentration and memory, as well as recurrent night-time awakenings.

Typically, the diagnostic process involves a comprehensive sleep study, known as polysomnography, which meticulously monitors various sleep parameters including breathing patterns, oxygen levels, and brain activity. In certain scenarios, home sleep tests may be employed to diagnose sleep apnea, offering a convenient alternative for some individuals.

The spectrum of treatment for sleep apnea encompasses lifestyle adjustments, including weight management, smoking cessation, and the avoidance of alcohol and sedatives. A notable therapeutic approach is Continuous Positive Airway Pressure (CPAP) therapy, involving a machine that administers pressurised air to sustain open airways during sleep. Oral appliances, strategically repositioning the jaw and tongue to prevent airway blockage, also offer a viable intervention. In severe cases, surgical options may be contemplated as part of the treatment plan.

Restless Leg Syndrome (RLS) is characterised by an irresistible urge to move the legs, frequently accompanied by uncomfortable sensations like tingling, crawling, or aching. These symptoms tend to intensify during the night or when resting, posing challenges in falling asleep or maintaining sleep. Movement or stretching of the legs often provides relief from these sensations.

Diagnosis primarily hinges on a clinical evaluation and the patient's detailed description of symptoms. In certain cases, diagnostic tools such as nocturnal polysomnography or actigraphy may be employed to exclude other sleep disorders or monitor disruptions in sleep attributed to RLS.

Addressing Restless Leg Syndrome (RLS) encompasses a range of interventions, starting with lifestyle adjustments like incorporating regular exercise and abstaining from caffeine and alcohol. Medications, including dopaminergic agents, opioids, or anticonvulsants, may be prescribed to alleviate symptoms. In instances where a deficiency is identified, iron supplementation becomes a consideration. Additionally, behavioural therapy and relaxation techniques serve as valuable tools in managing and mitigating RLS symptoms.

It's crucial to acknowledge that the manifestation of sleep disorders can differ from person to person, and the strategies for treatment may vary based on the severity and root causes. If you suspect the presence of a sleep disorder, seeking medical advice is prudent. Consultation with a healthcare provider or a specialised sleep expert can facilitate an accurate diagnosis and the formulation of a personalised treatment plan. Recognising the pivotal role of quality sleep in overall health and well-being and addressing sleep disorders can pave the way for substantial enhancements in one's life.

The interplay between diet, nutrition, sleep quality, and stress management are integral. The choices you make in what you eat, and drink wield significant influence over your ability to initiate and maintain sleep, as well as effectively manage stress.

Caffeine, a common component in coffee, tea, energy drinks, and certain sodas, operate as stimulants capable of disrupting sleep. By blocking the action of adenosine, a neurotransmitter that fosters sleep and relaxation, caffeine can impede the natural sleep-inducing processes. Therefore, it is advisable to steer clear of caffeine in the later parts of the day, as its presence can disrupt the circadian rhythm and pose challenges in the initiation of sleep.

Despite its initial sedative effects and the illusion of inducing drowsiness, alcohol proves to be a disruptor of the sleep cycle. It diminishes the duration of rejuvenating REM (rapid eye movement) sleep and contributes to fragmented sleep patterns. To enhance sleep quality, it is advisable to curtail alcohol consumption, especially in proximity to bedtime.

The consumption of heavy or spicy meals before retiring for the night carries the potential for indigestion and discomfort, thereby complicating the quest for restful sleep. Similarly, the intake of foods high in sugar can prompt fluctuations in blood sugar levels, leading to nocturnal awakenings. Prioritising light, easily digestible, and well-balanced meals can provide support for a more conducive sleep environment.

The repercussions of dehydration extend to dry mouth and nasal passages, potentially instigating snoring, and interrupting sleep. Although maintaining hydration is crucial, it's prudent to moderate fluid intake, especially in the moments preceding bedtime, to mitigate the likelihood of night-time awakenings for bathroom visits. Conversely, indulging in sizable or heavy meals near bedtime may result in discomfort and indigestion.

To foster optimal digestion and sleep quality, it is recommended to allow a gap of at least 2-3 hours between your last meal and bedtime. Yet, retiring to bed with a hungry stomach can also impede sleep quality. In such cases, a light and balanced snack may prove beneficial if hunger strikes before bedtime.

Specific vitamins and minerals, including B vitamins, vitamin C, and magnesium, assume a vital role in the realm of stress management. These nutrients actively participate in the body's stress response and contribute to the regulation of stress hormones. Ensuring a balanced diet rich in a variety of fruits, vegetables, and whole grains becomes pivotal to secure these essential elements.

Moreover, the inclusion of Omega-3 fatty acids, prevalent in fatty fish such as salmon and flaxseeds, can potentially aid in stress and anxiety reduction. Beyond their nutritional value, these fatty acids boast anti-inflammatory properties, offering benefits to both physical and mental well-being.

Fluctuations in blood sugar levels can contribute to both stress and mood swings. A stabilising approach involves the consumption of complex carbohydrates, high-fibre foods, and well-balanced meals to maintain blood sugar stability. Dehydration, on the other hand, can intensify the body's stress response, heightening feelings of anxiety and irritability. Therefore, prioritising adequate hydration is imperative for effective stress management.

The impact of highly processed foods and those laden with added sugars should not be overlooked, as they can induce spikes and crashes in blood sugar levels, thereby contributing to stress and mood fluctuations. Opting for a diet rich in whole, unprocessed foods generally aligns more favourably with effective stress management practices.

Consistent physical activity assumes a pivotal role in fostering improved sleep and diminishing stress. Exercise directly influences a spectrum of physiological and psychological factors that shape both sleep quality and stress levels. Engaging in regular physical activity, irrespective of the time of day, yields long-term enhancements in sleep quality.

It's worth noting that the timing of exercise can yield varied effects on individuals. Morning or afternoon exercise typically elevates body temperature, and the subsequent decline in temperature during the evening can contribute to promoting sleep.

However, evening exercise might prove overly invigorating for some individuals, potentially impeding the ability to initiate sleep. For those opting for evening workouts, the recommendation is to conclude the exercise routine at least 2-3 hours before bedtime, allowing the body temperature to gradually cool down. Aerobic exercises, such as running, swimming, or cycling, have demonstrated a positive influence on sleep quality, reducing the time taken to fall asleep and enhancing the duration of deep sleep.

Incorporating resistance training, including weightlifting, into one's routine can also contribute to improved sleep. This form of exercise not only enhances overall sleep quality but also diminishes the frequency of night-time awakenings. Furthermore, mind-body exercises like yoga and tai chi offer additional benefits by enhancing sleep quality and alleviating symptoms associated with insomnia.

Consistent exercise, undertaken on most days in the week, yields the most substantial influence on both the quality and duration of sleep. The recommended guideline for adults entails engaging in at least 150 minutes of moderate-intensity aerobic exercise or 75 minutes of vigorous-intensity aerobic exercise weekly, complemented by muscle strengthening activities on two or more days.

The ac of physical activity serves as a catalyst for the release of endorphins, the body's innate mood elevators. This mechanism contributes to the reduction of stress, anxiety, and depression. Beyond its direct impact on mental well-being, regular exercise elevates self-esteem, refines cognitive function, and imparts a sense of accomplishment, all of which collectively bolster effective stress management.

Aerobic exercises, ranging from running and brisk walking to dancing, prove effective in stress reduction by triggering the release of endorphins and enhancing overall well-being. Mind-body exercises like yoga and tai chi uniquely blend physical activity with relaxation and mindfulness techniques, rendering them particularly advantageous for stress alleviation.

Engaging in regular physical activity emerges as a proactive and positive coping mechanism for navigating stress. It acts as an outlet for both emotional and physical tension, fostering a balanced mental state. The involvement in group sports, outdoor activities, or team-based exercises introduces a social dimension that provides interaction and support, thereby further enhancing the effectiveness of stress reduction efforts.

Consistent engagement in physical activity presents a plethora of advantages for both sleep quality and stress reduction. The timing, nature of exercises, and the steadfastness of physical activity routines all merit consideration. Discovering an exercise regimen tailored to individual preferences and requirements enhances the prospect of sustaining a healthy and active lifestyle conducive to improved sleep and adept stress management.

Prior to embarking on a new exercise program, particularly if underlying health concerns exist, it is imperative to seek guidance from a healthcare professional or fitness expert. This precautionary step ensures that chosen exercise routines align seamlessly with health needs and goals.

Within an athlete's training and performance regimen, sleep and recovery assume integral roles. The calibre and duration of an athlete's sleep, along with the approaches employed for recovery, wield substantial influence over their physical and mental well-being, ultimately shaping their overall performance.

Delving into the significance of sleep and recovery for athletes, a comprehensive understanding unfolds. In the profound stages of deep sleep, the body releases growth hormones, an indispensable factor for muscle repair and growth. This recovery phase becomes paramount for athletes, offering the necessary time to mend the microtears in their muscles induced by training sessions.

The replenishment of glycogen stores, vital for energy in physical endeavours, particularly in endurance sports is a key function facilitated by sleep. In the absence of sufficient sleep, athletes may encounter premature fatigue during workouts or competitions. Beyond the physical aspect, sleep assumes a pivotal role in cognitive functions such as memory, decision-making, and reaction time, critical skills for sports demanding strategic thinking, coordination, and swift responses.

Maintaining a consistent sleep schedule contributes to the regulation of hormones, including cortisol and testosterone. This hormonal balance significantly influences an athlete's overall performance, mood, and recovery process. Therefore, prioritising adequate and regular sleep becomes a cornerstone in optimising an athlete's physical and mental capabilities.

Athletes, especially those immersed in demanding training regimens, may encounter a transient compromise in their immune system's resilience. Sufficient sleep emerges as a crucial factor in fortifying the immune system, thereby mitigating the susceptibility to illnesses or injuries that could impede training and competition.

Sleep stands at the forefront of stress reduction and recovery, essential elements for athletes navigating intensive training and competitive arenas. The accumulation of physical and mental stress during such endeavours finds alleviation through quality sleep, creating an environment conducive to the body's repair and regeneration.

For athletes committed to prioritising sleep, the dividends include an enhancement in performance metrics, ranging from improved speed and endurance to heightened accuracy and overall physical and mental capabilities. Additionally, the consolidation of motor skills and muscle memory is fostered by the restorative powers of sleep, contributing to a comprehensive elevation of athletic prowess.

Scheduled rest days are imperative for athletes, providing the necessary time for complete physical recovery. During these intervals, activities such as reduced-intensity training, stretching, and ensuring ample sleep become integral components. Incorporating active recovery techniques, such as swimming, cycling, or yoga proves beneficial for muscle relaxation and overall well-being.

The significance of proper post-workout nutrition cannot be overstated in the recovery process. A well-balanced intake of carbohydrates, proteins, and fats plays a pivotal role in replenishing energy stores and facilitating the repair of muscle tissue. Equally crucial is staying well-hydrated, as dehydration can impede the body's ability to effectively heal and repair. These mindful practices collectively contribute to an integrated approach to recovery.

Chapter 7 - Supercharging Your Immune System: Boosting Longevity Naturally

In an age where the spotlight is firmly on health and well-being, the pursuit of a resilient immune system has risen to prominence. Amidst a dynamic backdrop of evolving health concerns, the importance of reinforcing our body's innate defence mechanisms cannot be emphasised enough.

This chapter initiates a thorough exploration of strategies designed to help empower one's immune system, a comprehensive approach that not only safeguards against illnesses but also aligns with the overarching goal of achieving longevity through natural means.

We will intricately explore the workings of the immune system, unravelling its complexities and revealing the pivotal role it assumes in our holistic health. From grasping the foundational principles of immune function to delving into the symbiotic relationship connecting nutrition, lifestyle habits, and immune health, this journey empowers one to seize control of health and well-being.

Steered by the tenets of natural health improvement, we will navigate the landscape of evidence supported practices with the potential to enhance longevity. Nutrition stands as a cornerstone, with a meticulous examination of immune-boosting foods and dietary patterns. We will accurately analyse the influence of lifestyle choices, revealing habits that can either strengthen or compromise our body's inherent defence mechanisms.

Acknowledging the inseparable connection between physical activity and immune resilience, we will methodically examine the pivotal role of exercise in the quest for a strong immune system. Emphasising stress management, we will delve into the complex relationship between mental well-being and immune function.

Furthermore, we will unravel the vital significance that quality sleep assumes in this narrative, positioning it not merely as a foundation of immune support but also as a fundamental contributor to longevity.

Directing attention to environmental factors, their impact on immune health should be recognised. As we navigate through these dimensions, the incorporation of longevity practices emerges as a guiding principle, intricately weaving together diverse threads into a cohesive strategy aimed at fortifying our natural defences.

This chapter serves as a roadmap for those eager to embrace a holistic approach to health, one that not only safeguards against illnesses but also champions the journey towards a longer, healthier life through natural and sustainable means.

The immune system is an intricate and highly orchestrated network within the human body, acting as a formidable defence mechanism against a myriad of pathogens and foreign invaders. This is the body's first line of defence, a rapid and generic response to any foreign substance. Components like physical barriers (skin and mucous membranes) and cells such as macrophages and neutrophils play pivotal roles in this immediate defence.

In the realm of the immune system, precision reigns supreme as the immune system unveils its highly specialised prowess tailored to specific pathogens. At the forefront of adaptive immunity, T and B lymphocytes emerge as the principal protagonists, adeptly committing past encounters with pathogens to memory. This meticulous recollection sets the stage for a rapid and precisely targeted response upon subsequent exposure.

A marvel of nature, the immune system exhibits a remarkable capacity for distinguishing between "self" and "non-self." This inherent ability acts as a vigilant guardian, ensuring that its focus remains solely on foreign substances, thereby safeguarding the body from any inadvertent assault on its own cells.

Employing a sophisticated array of mechanisms, the immune system orchestrates a symphony of defence. It unleashes the arsenal of antibodies, engages in the art of phagocytosis to engulf invaders, and activates complement proteins, all in a choreographed effort to neutralise and eliminate pathogens with unwavering efficiency.

In a testament to its extraordinary capabilities, the immune system possesses the remarkable ability to retain a memory of past encounters with pathogens. This recollection, orchestrated by the intricate interplay of T and B cells, sets the stage for a swifter and more formidable response upon encountering the same threat again.

The vitality of an efficiently operating immune system is paramount to sustaining optimal health. Beyond its role in warding off infectious agents, this intricate defence mechanism assumes a critical role in diligently monitoring and eradicating aberrant cells within the body, including those with the potential to instigate cancer.

Optimal nutrition, with a focus on a balanced intake of essential vitamins and minerals, stands as a cornerstone for the effective operation of the immune system. Specific nutrients, including vitamin C, vitamin D, and zinc, assume distinct roles in supporting immune function.

Beyond nutrition, lifestyle factors such as regular exercise, ample sleep, and effective stress management wield considerable influence over immune health.

For instance, exercise has the potential to enhance the circulation of immune cells, while persistent stress may exert immunosuppressive effects. As the sands of time shift, the immune system, too, undergoes changes, exhibiting a propensity for functional decline with age. Recognising these age-related alterations becomes pivotal in tailoring targeted immune support strategies that align with the distinct needs of various life stages.

In the quest for enduring well-being, the emphasis lies in fortifying the innate defence mechanisms of the body. There is an array of natural strategies meticulously crafted to enhance immunity, such as nutritional methodologies, lifestyle adjustments, and integrative approaches that foster the robustness of the immune system.

The inclusion of antioxidant-rich foods, notably fruits and vegetables, assumes a pivotal role in quelling free radicals and nurturing immune functionality. Notably, vitamins C and E, alongside minerals such as selenium and zinc, emerge as particularly vital components in this intricate tapestry of immune support.

The gastrointestinal tract harbours a substantial segment of the immune system. Probiotics, inherent in fermented delicacies like yogurt and kefir, play a pivotal role in cultivating a thriving gut microbiome, thereby exerting a positive influence on immune responses. The maintenance of adequate vitamin D levels is intricately linked to fortified immune function. This can be achieved through a combination of sun exposure, dietary sources like fatty fish, and supplementation if required, ensuring the sustenance of optimal vitamin D levels.

In the realm of traditional wellness, certain herbs, including echinacea, elderberry, and astragalus, have been time-honoured for their role in bolstering immune function. These botanical wonders highlight immune-modulating properties, contributing to the intricate interplay of the body's defence mechanisms.

The influence of physical activity on immune function is profound. Consistent, moderate exercise is linked to an enhanced circulation of immune cells, mitigating the vulnerability to infections. Essential to immune health is the foundation of quality sleep. In the realm of slumber, the body engages in pivotal processes, releasing cytokines that play a vital role in supporting immune function.

Conversely, chronic stress poses a threat to immune function. Adopting practices like mindfulness, meditation, and yoga can function as potent antidotes to stress, fostering a more resilient immune system. Acupuncture and the principles of Traditional Chinese Medicine are thought to recalibrate the body's energy flow, providing support to immune function.

Homeopathic remedies are sought by some to invigorate the body's vital force and address underlying imbalances that may impact immunity. The time-honoured system of Ayurveda integrates herbs, dietary guidance, and lifestyle practices to foster harmony within the body, promoting not only overall well-being but also immune health.

In the realm of practical measures, the straightforward yet impactful practices of regular handwashing and maintaining good hygiene serve as effective safeguards against the spread of infections. These habits alleviate the burden on the immune system, underlining the importance of simple yet conscientious actions in bolstering our body's defence mechanisms. Minimising exposure to environmental pollutants and toxins plays a pivotal role in nurturing comprehensive immune health.

At the core of upholding a robust immune system is the intricate connection between nutrition and immune health. Recognised for its potent antioxidant properties, vitamin C assumes a critical role in the production and functionality of white blood cells.

Excellent sources of this vital nutrient include citrus fruits, strawberries, and bell peppers. Another key player in immune response modulation is vitamin D, synthesised in the skin through exposure to sunlight. Sustaining optimal levels can be achieved through the consumption of fatty fish, fortified dairy products, and, if necessary, supplementation.

Zinc, with its immune cell support and antiviral properties, can be obtained from sources such as meat, dairy, nuts, and legumes. Amino acids derived from protein sources play a crucial role in the synthesis of antibodies and immune cells, and this role is fulfilled by lean meats, poultry, fish, and plant-based proteins.

Iron, essential for the proliferation of immune cells, is found in abundance in lean meats, beans, lentils, and fortified cereals. Probiotics, present in fermented foods like yogurt, kefir, and sauerkraut, contribute to a healthy gut microbiome, influencing immune responses positively.

Berries such as blueberries, strawberries, and raspberries stand out for their antioxidant richness, actively combatting oxidative stress and bolstering immune cells. Leafy greens like spinach and kale offer a wealth of vitamins and minerals, making a substantial contribution to overall immune function.

Nutrient-dense options like almonds, sunflower seeds, and walnuts provide a mix of vitamin E, zinc, and healthy fats, promoting optimal immune health. Carrots, sweet potatoes, and bell peppers, rich in beta-carotene, serve as precursors to vitamin A, further supporting immune function.

Salmon, mackerel, and trout boast elevated levels of omega-3 fatty acids, renowned for their anti-inflammatory properties that have a positive impact on immune responses. Plant-based sources of omega-3 fatty acids play a role in maintaining a balanced and anti-inflammatory diet. The Mediterranean diet, centred around an emphasis on fruits, vegetables, whole grains, and healthy fats, offers a diverse array of nutrients that actively support immune function.

The Dietary Approaches to Stop Hypertension (DASH) diet, featuring an abundance of fruits, vegetables, lean proteins, and low-fat dairy, actively contributes to overall health and immune support. Maintaining proper hydration is crucial for optimal immune function, as water facilitates nutrient transport and waste elimination.

Excessive sugar intake can compromise immune function, underscoring the importance of a balanced and diverse diet that avoids excessive processed foods. Recognising that dietary needs can vary based on factors such as age, health conditions, and lifestyle, the significance of tailoring nutritional choices to individual requirements cannot be overstated.

Grasping the intricate link between nutrition and immune health empowers individuals to make well-informed dietary choices that enhance the resilience of their immune system. This integrated approach, when combined with a balanced lifestyle, becomes a foundational element in cultivating overall well-being and immune vitality.

Preserving a resilient immune system is pivotal for holistic health and well-being. Numerous lifestyle habits play a role in supporting and fortifying the immune system. Incorporating a diverse range of fruits, vegetables, whole grains, lean proteins, and healthy fats into your diet is essential.

Prioritise foods abundant in essential vitamins and minerals, including vitamin C, vitamin D, zinc, and antioxidants. Additionally, consider integrating probiotics from fermented foods like yogurt and kefir to foster a healthy gut, thus positively influencing immune function.

Maintaining proper hydration is paramount for overall health and plays a pivotal role in supporting immune system function. Adequate water intake facilitates the flushing of toxins from the body and ensures the smooth operation of various physiological processes. Engaging in moderate and regular physical activity is strongly associated with enhanced immune function. Exercise promotes optimal circulation, enabling immune cells to move freely throughout the body.

Strive for 7-9 hours of restorative sleep each night to facilitate the body's repair and regeneration processes. Insufficient sleep can compromise the immune system, increasing vulnerability to infections. Chronic stress has a detrimental effect on immune function. Integrate stress-reducing practices like meditation, yoga, deep breathing, or mindfulness into your routine. Prioritise time for relaxation and engage in hobbies to alleviate daily stressors. Regularly wash your hands with soap and water to prevent the spread of infections.

Avoid touching your face, particularly the eyes, nose, and mouth, to minimise the risk of introducing pathogens into the body. Excessive alcohol consumption can compromise the immune system, thus, it's advisable to consume alcohol in moderation or consider abstaining altogether.

Smoking poses harm to the respiratory system and weakens the immune system. Quitting smoking can yield substantial benefits for overall health. Obesity has been associated with impaired immune function, underscoring the importance of adopting a healthy lifestyle that encompasses a balanced diet and regular exercise to maintain a healthy weight.

Cultivate and nurture social connections with friends and family, recognising that strong social ties are correlated with enhanced immune function. Positive social interactions play a pivotal role in promoting overall emotional well-being. Ensure you stay current with vaccinations, as they offer crucial protection against specific infectious diseases.

Keep in mind that individual responses to lifestyle changes can differ, emphasising the importance of consulting healthcare professionals for personalised advice, particularly if you have underlying health conditions or concerns about your immune system. Implementing a combination of these habits forms a comprehensive approach to supporting the immune system.

Physical exercise holds a pivotal role in sustaining a robust immune system. Consistent physical activity has demonstrated a myriad of positive effects on the immune system, fostering overall well-being and mitigating the risk of illness. Exercise enhances blood circulation, facilitating the more efficient movement of immune cells throughout the body.

This improved circulation aids in the transportation of immune cells and antibodies to sites of infection or inflammation. Furthermore, regular exercise exhibits anti-inflammatory effects, contributing to the reduction of chronic inflammation.

Chronic inflammation is intricately connected to various health issues, potentially compromising immune function. Exercise serves as a catalyst to produce diverse immune cells, including white blood cells and natural killer cells. These cells assume a pivotal role in identifying and eliminating pathogens like viruses and bacteria.

Moderate-intensity exercise has been correlated with an uptick in antibody production, thereby augmenting the body's capacity to combat infections. Engaging in regular, moderate exercise positively influences the adaptive immune system.

Chronic stress has the potential to weaken the immune system, but exercise emerges as a natural stress reliever. It stimulates the release of endorphins and reduces stress hormones, fostering an environment conducive to stress reduction. This, in turn, contributes to the fortification of a more resilient immune system.

Specifically, aerobic exercise bolsters the respiratory system, enhancing its function and, consequently, reinforcing the body's defence against respiratory infections. Additionally, exercise plays a crucial role in regulating the body's inflammatory response, preventing it from becoming excessive or chronic. This proper regulation of inflammation is pivotal for maintaining the delicate balance of the immune system.

Engaging in physical activity exerts a positive influence on the gut microbiota, a pivotal player in the regulation of the immune system. The cultivation of a healthy gut microbiome, in turn, contributes significantly to the overall functionality of the immune system.

The enduring benefits of immune health are bestowed upon those who embrace a regimen of regular and consistent exercise. However, it is imperative to tread the path of balance, as overtraining or subjecting oneself to intense physical exertion without adequate recovery may yield adverse effects.

Noteworthy is the capacity of exercise to assuage the age-related decline in immune function. Among older adults, a commitment to regular physical activity often manifests in improved immune responses. Thus, the integration of a well-rounded and sustainable exercise routine emerges as a cornerstone in fortifying the intricate relationship between physical activity and immune vitality.

While moderate exercise typically yields overall benefits, it's crucial to note that excessively intense or prolonged physical activity might transiently hinder the immune system. Athletes, therefore, should conscientiously consider strategies for recovery and immune support. The impact of exercise on the immune system exhibits variability among individuals, with factors such as age, fitness level, and overall health influencing responses.

The incorporation of regular, moderate exercise into one's routine emerges as a significant contributor to maintaining a robust immune system. Striking a balance tailored to your fitness level and overall health becomes essential. Prior to making substantial alterations to your exercise regimen, particularly if you harbour underlying health concerns, it is prudent to seek guidance from healthcare professionals. Their expertise ensures a thoughtful approach to safeguarding your health and well-being.

Maintaining a resilient immune system is contingent upon effective stress management. The ramifications of chronic stress can detrimentally affect the immune response, rendering the body more susceptible to infections and various health issues. A particularly efficacious method for stress reduction is mindfulness meditation, which entails concentrating on the present moment without passing judgment.

Scientifically validated, this practice not only alleviates stress but also enhances immune function. The adoption of mindfulness practices has demonstrated the potential to diminish inflammatory markers and augment the activity of natural killer cells, underscoring its significance in fortifying the immune system.

Engaging in diaphragmatic breathing, box breathing, and various deep breathing exercises triggers the body's relaxation response. This intentional focus on deep breathing effectively diminishes stress hormones, fostering a state of relaxation that distinctly benefits the immune system.

Another valuable relaxation technique is Progressive Muscle Relaxation (PMR), wherein muscle groups are alternately tensed and then released. This practice not only promotes physical and mental relaxation but also contributes to a reduction in overall stress levels, potentially enhancing immune function.

Yoga seamlessly integrates physical postures, breath control, and meditation, offering a comprehensive strategy for managing stress. Consistent engagement in yoga has been correlated with decreased stress and inflammation levels. Through physical activity, yoga stimulates the release of endorphins, the body's innate mood elevators.

The incorporation of regular, moderate exercise, including yoga, not only diminishes stress but also bolsters overall immune system health. In addition to physical practices, fostering robust social connections proves instrumental in garnering emotional support amidst challenging periods. Positive social interactions are intricately tied to an enhanced immune response, underscoring the holistic benefits of maintaining strong social bonds.

Cognitive-Behavioural Therapy (CBT) empowers individuals to recognise and modify negative thought patterns and behaviours. This therapeutic approach has shown a correlation with diminished stress and enhanced immune function. Skilful time management and prioritisation contribute to a reduction in feelings of overwhelm and stress, consequently exerting a positive influence on the immune system. Effectively managing chronic stressors is crucial for nurturing overall well-being.

On a lighter note, the simple act of laughter acts as a natural catalyst for the release of endorphins, fostering a deep sense of well-being. Notably, scientific research has established a connection between laughter and improved immune responses, underscoring its therapeutic role in sustaining immune vitality.

Participating in activities that bring you joy offers a valuable mental respite and diminishes stress. Hobbies and leisure pursuits play a role in fostering a positive mood, thereby contributing to the well-being of the immune system. During stressful periods, it's advisable to limit caffeine and alcohol intake. The overconsumption of stimulants can escalate stress levels, disrupt sleep, and adversely affect immune health.

Integrating a combination of stress management techniques into your lifestyle can yield a positive impact on immune function. It's essential to identify strategies that resonate with you and to maintain consistency in their practice. If stress becomes chronic or overwhelming, seeking support from healthcare professionals or mental health experts is a prudent course of action.

High-quality sleep stands as a crucial cornerstone in bolstering immune support, playing an indispensable role in sustaining overall health and well-being. Throughout the sleep cycle, the body undergoes vital processes that contribute to immune function, tissue repair, and comprehensive physical and mental resilience. Comprising various stages, including REM (Rapid Eye Movement) and non-REM phases, each segment serves a distinct purpose in the realm of physiological restoration.

The influence of sleep extends to the production of cytokines, pivotal proteins that orchestrate immune responses. During the phases of deep sleep, immune cells such as T cells and cytokines exhibit heightened activity, fortifying the body's defence mechanisms against infections. In essence, the profound impact of quality sleep on immune vitality underscores its significance in the broader landscape of health maintenance.

Sufficient sleep plays a crucial role in regulating the body's inflammatory response. Insufficient sleep, on the other hand, may contribute to chronic low-grade inflammation, linked to a range of health issues. During deep sleep, the body releases growth hormones, facilitating cellular repair and regeneration. This highlights the importance of quality sleep in the healing and restoration of tissues, especially those integral to immune responses.

Beyond its impact on physical health, sleep is paramount for cognitive functions such as memory consolidation and learning. A well-rested brain supports effective communication between the nervous and immune systems, emphasising the complex connection between restorative sleep and overall well-rounded health.

Melatonin, a hormone generated during sleep, boasts antioxidant properties, and actively participates in the regulation of the sleep-wake cycle. Beyond its role in facilitating a restful night, melatonin may also exert influence on immune function, aiding the body in its response to infections.

It is crucial to acknowledge that chronic sleep deprivation has the potential to compromise the immune response, rendering the body more susceptible to infections. Thus, prioritising a sufficient and regular sleep routine emerges as a fundamental aspect of maintaining robust immune health.

Lack of sleep is associated with increased inflammation and a higher risk of chronic conditions. Aligning sleep patterns with natural circadian rhythms promotes better sleep quality. Properly timed sleep supports the balance of hormones, including those related to stress and immunity.

Create a comfortable, dark, and quiet sleep environment. Limit exposure to screens before bedtime to promote the natural production of melatonin. Establishing a calming routine before bedtime signals the body that it's time to sleep.

The sophisticated relationship between quality sleep and stress management unveils a profound connection. Sufficient sleep not only fortifies resilience against stressors but also fosters holistic well-being. Persistent sleep disorders warrant attention from healthcare professionals for precise diagnosis and effective treatment.

The significance of identifying and rectifying sleep disorders extends to the realm of immune health. Indeed, quality sleep stands as a cornerstone for a robust immune system. Cultivating good sleep hygiene, forging consistent sleep patterns, and attending to sleep-related concerns collectively contribute to comprehensive immune support. In cases where sleep-related issues endure, seeking guidance from healthcare professionals becomes prudent, ensuring a thorough safeguarding of immune health.

The vitality of immune health is meticulously intertwined with environmental factors, casting a substantial influence on individuals' well-being. The places where we dwell, toil, and engage in our daily activities wield a palpable sway over the efficacy and adaptability of our immune system. Subpar air quality, characterised by heightened levels of pollutants, can impart deleterious effects on respiratory wellness. The exposure to such airborne pollutants not only amplifies susceptibility to respiratory infections but also worsens pre-existing respiratory ailments.

Sufficient exposure to a variety of microbes in the environment during early childhood is linked to a stronger immune system. The immune function is shaped by the diversity and equilibrium of the microbiome, which, in turn, is influenced by environmental factors. Sunlight exposure contributes to the body's synthesis of vitamin D, a crucial element for immune health.

Alterations in temperature and humidity can influence the transmission and potency of specific infectious agents. Consumption of water tainted with pollutants or pathogens can impact gastrointestinal health and, consequently, the immune system. Adequate hydration is imperative for holistic well-being and sustains diverse physiological processes, including immune function.

Residence in urban or rural settings can shape the encounter with pollutants, allergens, and infectious agents, subsequently influencing immune responses. Proximity to green spaces and nature correlates with beneficial effects on both mental and physical well-being, potentially exerting an impact on immune function.

Specific occupational exposures, such as those involving chemicals or pollutants, may have repercussions on respiratory and immune health. Irregular work schedules, particularly night shifts, have the potential to disrupt circadian rhythms, thereby affecting immune function. Encountering allergens has the potential to initiate allergic reactions, impacting both respiratory and immune responses. The quality of one's diet, encompassing the intake of nutrients and antioxidants, plays a pivotal role in influencing immune function.

Food that is contaminated or mishandled poses a risk of infections, placing a challenge on the immune system. Practices related to hygiene, such as thorough handwashing and sanitation, influences the dissemination of infectious agents. Overcrowded environments can create conditions conducive to the transmission of infectious diseases.

Persistent stress, whether originating from work, relationships, or other sources, has the potential to influence immune function. The adoption of healthy coping mechanisms and effective stress management becomes imperative for sustaining immune resilience.

Contact with environmental toxins, including heavy metals or industrial chemicals, can induce immunotoxin effects. Specific chemicals may interfere with the endocrine system, thereby impacting immune function. Discrepancies in access to healthcare services can significantly impact an individual's capacity to prevent, diagnose, and manage health conditions that affect the immune system.

The vaccination policies implemented within a community wield a profound influence on establishing herd immunity, safeguarding vulnerable individuals, and alleviating the collective burden of infectious diseases. The complex dynamics of immune health are shaped by a myriad of environmental factors. The interplay among genetics, lifestyle choices, and the external environment underscores the sophisticated regulation of the immune system.

Initiatives geared towards promoting immune health ought to consider these environmental factors, striving to cultivate conditions conducive to a robust and adaptable immune system. Furthermore, public health measures and policies play a pivotal role in creating environments that nurture community well-being and fortify immune resilience.

Incorporating longevity practices entails adopting lifestyle habits and strategies with the aim of enhancing overall health and well-being, ultimately seeking to extend both the quality and duration of life. Longevity practices often encompass facets related to physical, mental, and social well-being.

Certain studies suggest that reducing calorie intake without compromising nutrition may offer potential benefits for longevity and age-related diseases. This involves restricting the daily eating window, potentially fostering metabolic health and cellular repair. Prolonged periods of fasting or alternate day fasting may exhibit positive effects on pathways associated with longevity. These practices contribute to the improvement of cardiovascular health and overall fitness, while also aiding in the maintenance of muscle mass and bone density, crucial components for ageing well.

Promote mobility and minimise the risk of falls, particularly among older adults. Embrace practices that foster relaxation, diminish stress hormones, and bolster mental well-being. Integrate physical postures, breath control, and meditation to foster stress reduction and enhance overall health. Enhance both physical and mental well-being, encompassing immune function, memory consolidation, and hormonal equilibrium. Establish a regular sleep routine and cultivate an environment conducive to restful sleep.

Cultivate meaningful social connections and actively engage in social pursuits. The presence of a robust support system is associated with improved mental well-being and increased longevity. Challenge the mind through activities like solving puzzles, acquiring new skills, and pursuing hobbies. Foster a commitment to ongoing learning and seek intellectual stimulation. Minimise or abstain from smoking and excessive alcohol consumption. Refrain from the misuse of prescription or recreational drugs.

Adhere to routine health check-ups and screenings tailored to age-related diseases. Keep current with vaccinations to thwart infectious diseases. Consider individual genetic factors when managing health. Delve into lifestyle practices that potentially positively impact gene expression. Reduce exposure to pollutants, toxins, and harmful chemicals. Embrace green spaces and forge a connection with nature. Cultivate a positive outlook and resilience in confronting challenges. Centre attention on gratitude and an appreciation for life.

Participate in activities that harmonise spiritual and mental well-being. Cultivate a sense of purpose and meaning in life. Integrate complementary and alternative therapies into your healthcare regimen. Customise healthcare strategies according to individual health profiles.

The integration of longevity practices adopts a comprehensive health approach, addressing physical, mental, and social well-being. These practices are not isolated but interlinked, and their combined effects contribute to a richer and more satisfying life. It's crucial to recognise that individual needs may differ and seeking personalised advice from healthcare professionals is advisable when contemplating substantial lifestyle changes.

Recognising the dynamic nature of life, the inclusion of seasonal adjustments in dietary choices and lifestyle practices adds a layer of adaptability to the pursuit of immune resilience. Acknowledging and addressing the changing needs of the body throughout the seasons is a key aspect of a sustainable health journey. In the pursuit of supercharging the immune system for enhanced longevity, it is crucial to view health as a lifelong journey rather than a destination.

Chapter 8 - Harnessing the Benefits of Mindfulness and Meditation

Mindfulness, a cognitive state distinguished by heightened awareness and an unwavering focus on the present moment devoid of judgment, is a practice rooted in ancient contemplative traditions, notably within the realm of Buddhism. Its essence, however, transcends these origins, finding a contemporary and secularised application for widespread benefit. At its core, mindfulness entails a complete immersion in one's thoughts, emotions, and surroundings.

With origins traced back to the profound teachings of Buddhist traditions, mindfulness has evolved into a universal tool, accessible to individuals irrespective of their spiritual inclinations. The essence of this practice lies in the ability to be fully attuned to the current moment, allowing the unfurling of thoughts and sensations without the imposition of judgment. We must diligently foster a non-judgmental mindset, embracing thoughts and emotions without categorising them into the dichotomy of good or bad.

Central to the practice of mindfulness is the deliberate redirection of attention to a chosen focal point, whether it be the rhythmic cadence of breath, the subtle nuances of bodily sensations, or the contemplation of an external object. Through this intentional focus, individuals embark on a journey of heightened awareness, fostering a state of mindfulness that transcends the temporal constraints of past and future, anchoring them firmly in the richness of the present.

Mindfulness finds its intentional cultivation through the practice of meditation. Meditation serves as a deliberate means to foster and fortify mindfulness, functioning as a method or tool in this pursuit. One prominent application of mindfulness is found in Mindfulness-Based Stress Reduction (MBSR), a structured program that seamlessly weaves mindfulness meditation into its framework, aiming to alleviate stress and elevate overall well-being.

Another noteworthy approach is embodied in Mindfulness-Based Cognitive Therapy (MBCT), a methodology that intertwines mindfulness practices with cognitive therapy techniques. Specifically designed to thwart relapses in individuals grappling with recurrent depression, MBCT stands as a testament to the power of combining mindfulness and therapeutic strategies in fostering mental resilience.

Mindful Breathing serves as a foundational practice, directing one's focus to the breath and attentively observing inhalations and exhalations without attachment. The essence lies in the simplicity of this exercise, fostering a heightened awareness of the present moment through the rhythmic cadence of breathing.

The Body Scan, another integral practice, entails a systematic and deliberate attention to bodily sensations. This method facilitates an increased awareness of both tension and relaxation within the body, offering a nuanced exploration of one's physical state.

In Loving-Kindness Meditation, the scope of mindfulness expands beyond the self. This practice is dedicated to cultivating feelings of compassion and love, extending benevolence not only to oneself but also radiating towards others. It stands as a profound exploration of mindfulness, emphasising the interconnectedness of individuals and fostering a heartful presence in the world.

Engaging in mindfulness practices has the potential to bring about notable changes in both the structure and function of the brain, particularly in regions linked to attention and emotional regulation. A wealth of studies attests to the effectiveness of mindfulness in mitigating stress, amplifying cognitive function, and fostering an overall improvement in mental well-being.

In the realm of mindful eating, the act of paying complete attention to the sensory experience can serve as a catalyst for cultivating healthier eating habits. This deliberate focus on the textures, flavours, and sensations of each bite encourages a more mindful and balanced approach to nourishment.

Similarly, the intentional practice of walking with heightened awareness, mindful of each step and the surrounding environment, becomes a mindful endeavour. This simple act transcends mere physical movement, transforming into a contemplative practice that connects one intimately with the present moment.

Moreover, mindfulness plays a pivotal role in enhancing interpersonal relationships. By bringing full attention to conversations, individuals can foster deeper connections and richer understanding. This intentional presence in dialogue contributes significantly to the quality of relationships, creating a space for authentic and meaningful connections to flourish.

Mindfulness is complexly tied to enhanced emotional regulation, offering a buffer against the adverse effects of stressors on mental health. The regular incorporation of mindfulness into one's routine is associated with marked improvements in sustained attention and cognitive performance, showcasing its multifaceted benefits.

In the teachings of mindfulness, ethical considerations play a significant role, with an emphasis on principles such as compassion, non-harm, and ethical conduct. These guidelines serve as a compass, guiding individuals toward a mindful existence that extends beyond personal well-being to encompass a broader ethical framework.

The ubiquity of technology and constant connectivity presents formidable challenges to fostering mindfulness in a digitally dominated world. Navigating this landscape requires a nuanced understanding of how mindfulness can coexist with the demands of our technologically driven lives.

To grasp the essence of mindfulness, one must delve into its historical roots, fundamental principles, diverse array of practices, and its applications across various fields. This exploration is essential for appreciating the growing significance of mindfulness in contemporary society, a dynamic concept with the potential to positively influence mental well-being, cognitive function, and the overall quality of life.

Direct your focus to the rhythmic cadence of your breath, attentively observing each inhalation and exhalation. Engage in intentional, deep breathing, and consider counting each breath cycle or immersing yourself in the sensations accompanying each breath. Systematically guide your attention through various parts of the body, noting sensations without passing judgment. Embark on this journey from the toes upward, gradually encompassing awareness of each body part.

In the realm of cultivating mindfulness, extend feelings of love and compassion inward and outward. Utter phrases such as "May I/you be happy, may I/you be healthy," broadening the circle of well-wishing to include friends, family, and even those with whom you may find difficulties.

When walking, adopt a deliberate and unhurried pace, savouring each step and tuning into the sensations in your feet. Take this practice to the outdoors, engaging in mindful walking amidst nature. As you move, attentively observe the sights, sounds, and sensations that unfold with each step, fostering a profound connection with the surrounding environment.

Indulge in a deliberate and unhurried dining experience by savouring each bite, attuning your awareness to the taste, texture, and sensations. Designate a specific meal to partake in mindful eating, immersing yourself in the sensory delights while avoiding distractions. Incorporate mindfulness into your yoga practice by intertwining conscious breathing with your postures, creating a harmonious synchronisation of breath and movement. Consider attending a yoga class or following online sessions that emphasise the integration of mindful breath and purposeful movement.

Choose an object or scene and engage in focused observation, absorbing its details without passing judgment. Dedicate a few moments to contemplating a natural element, such as a flower or a scene in your surroundings, allowing your attention to linger on the intricate details. Practice active listening by fully immersing yourself in a conversation, withholding immediate responses or judgments. Give your undivided attention to the speaker's words and non-verbal cues, fostering a deep and meaningful exchange.

Partake in colouring activities with complete mindfulness, directing your attention to the colours, shapes, and the fluidity of your hand movements. Explore colouring books tailored for mindfulness or unleash your creativity by designing your own patterns. Infuse mindful breathing into your routine by pairing it with visualisations of serene scenes or affirmations. Inhale positive energy and exhale stress, envisioning a tranquil place or repeating a soothing mantra.

Establish deliberate time frames for engaging with technology, eschewing multitasking, and mindless scrolling. Practice mindful phone usage by dedicating your focus to one task at a time, punctuating your efforts with breaks for conscious breathing and resetting. Pause periodically throughout the day to connect with your emotions and physical sensations. Employ alarms or reminders to prompt brief breaks, allowing you to bring your awareness to the present state of your mind and body.

Capture your thoughts, feelings, and observations in writing, allowing them to unfold without the weight of judgment. Allocate a dedicated time each day to ponder your experiences and emotions, cultivating a profound sense of self-awareness. Delve into gratitude by reflecting on and expressing appreciation for the positive facets of your life. Chronicle these moments in a gratitude journal, acknowledging and recording the things you're thankful for each day.

Bring mindful awareness to transitions between activities or environments. Prior to embarking on a new task, afford yourself a moment to breathe and centre your focus, establishing a mindful connection with the present. Integrate a spectrum of mindfulness techniques and exercises into your daily routine, offering a diverse exploration to discover what resonates best with your preferences and needs. Regular practice serves as a steadfast ally in honing mindfulness skills, ultimately contributing to the enhancement of overall well-being.

Diverse meditation practices offer unique approaches and focal points. Mindfulness Meditation centres on cultivating awareness of the present moment by observing thoughts and sensations without attachment, often using the breath as a focal point. Loving-Kindness Meditation, also known as Metta, focuses on nurturing feelings of love and compassion. This practice involves repeating phrases to extend well-wishes and loving-kindness both to oneself and others.

In Transcendental Meditation (TM), the emphasis lies in silently repeating a mantra. The technique involves sitting with closed eyes, directing focus onto the mantra to facilitate a state of restful awareness. Each of these meditation styles provides a distinctive avenue for individuals to explore and cultivate mindfulness in their own way.

In Body Scan Meditation, the emphasis is on systematically scanning the body for sensations. This involves bringing awareness to each part of the body and noting sensations without passing judgment. Zen Meditation, or Zazen, centres on attention to both breath and posture. During seated meditation, typically in a specific posture, the focus is on the breath or an aspect of existence. Guided Meditation shifts the focus to directed mental imagery or visualisation. A guide leads participants through a series of images or scenarios designed to evoke relaxation or promote self-discovery.

Vipassana Meditation centres on gaining insight into the true nature of reality. This is achieved by observing bodily sensations, providing a pathway to understanding the impermanence and interconnectedness of our experiences. Chakra Meditation places its focus on aligning and balancing energy centres, known as chakras. Participants concentrate on each chakra through visualisation, breathwork, or chanting, fostering a sense of harmony within.

In Mantra Meditation, the emphasis is on the repetition of a specific word or phrase. By focusing on the mantra's repetition, individuals aim to quiet the mind and cultivate inner stillness. Each of these meditation practices offers a distinctive approach to exploring deeper aspects of self-awareness and mindfulness.

Yoga Nidra centres on inducing deep relaxation and a state akin to conscious sleep. This practice involves lying down in a comfortable position while being guided through a systematic relaxation of both the body and mind. Walking Meditation emphasises mindful movement and breath awareness. The key is to engage in slow and deliberate walking, attentively focusing on each step and breath, fostering a heightened awareness of the present moment.

Sound Bath Meditation immerses individuals in the vibrational resonance of various sounds, such as singing bowls or gongs. Through exposure to these sounds, participants experience a profound sense of relaxation and connection. Kundalini Meditation directs its focus towards awakening spiritual energy, known as kundalini. This involves a combination of breathwork, chanting, and movement designed to activate and balance energy centres within the body.

Qi Gong Meditation is dedicated to harmonising and amplifying the flow of life energy, known as Qi. This is achieved through a holistic approach that combines movement, breath, and visualisation, fostering overall well-being. Breath Awareness Meditation centres on the conscious control and observation of breath. By directing attention to the breath and keenly observing its natural flow and rhythm, participants engage in a meditative practice that promotes mindfulness.

Achieving effectiveness in meditation involves the thoughtful creation of a conducive environment, the adoption of a comfortable posture, and the cultivation of a consistent practice. Begin by selecting a quiet and comfortable space where interruptions are minimised. Consider incorporating soft lighting and maintaining a moderate room temperature to enhance the overall atmosphere.

Establishing a regular meditation schedule is paramount. Whether opting for a daily practice or a few times a week, the key lies in maintaining consistency. Choose a time that seamlessly fits into your routine, whether it be in the morning, during a break, or before bedtime. When assuming your meditation posture, either sitting or lying down, prioritise comfort.

If seated, employ a cushion or chair for additional support. Maintain a straight yet relaxed back and let your shoulders ease into a state of relaxation. Allow your hands to rest naturally on your lap or knees, creating a posture that encourages a sense of comfort and focus.

Commence your meditation by directing your attention to your breath. Observe the rhythm of inhalation and exhalation. Should your mind begin to stray, gently guide your focus back to the breath. Acknowledge that meditation is a skill to be honed, and it's entirely normal for the mind to wander. Exercise patience with yourself and refrain from self-judgment.

Explore diverse meditation techniques, such as mindfulness, loving-kindness, or guided meditation. Find a method that resonates with you and aligns with your objectives. Particularly if you are new to meditation, consider utilising guided meditation sessions. Numerous apps and online resources offer a wealth of guided sessions to facilitate your practice.

Initiate your practice with shorter sessions, perhaps starting at 5 to 10 minutes, and progressively extend the duration as you grow more at ease. Emphasise the quality of your meditation over its quantity, recognising that consistency holds more significance than the length of each session. Should tension arise during your practice, conduct a brief body scan. Direct your awareness to each part of your body and deliberately release any tension. If necessary, incorporate progressive muscle relaxation techniques.

Broaden your awareness beyond the breath to encompass sounds, sensations, and thoughts. Observe these elements without forming attachments or passing judgments. If sitting on the floor becomes uncomfortable, consider using props such as cushions or benches. Prioritise a relaxed and sustainable posture throughout the entirety of your session.

Ease in and out of meditation, avoid abrupt movements or rushing back into daily activities. Take a moment to transition mindfully, acknowledging the present moment. Gradually increase the complexity of your meditation practice as you become more comfortable. Explore advanced techniques or longer sessions when you feel ready. Be open to adapting your meditation practice to suit your evolving needs and circumstances.

Feel free to explore various approaches as you progress on your meditation journey. Consider attending meditation classes or workshops and seek guidance from seasoned practitioners. Engaging with meditation communities or online forums can offer valuable support and shared experiences.

Keep in mind that meditation is a personal journey, and there's no universally applicable approach. Embrace the opportunity to experiment with different techniques, exercise patience with yourself, and relish the process of self-discovery and the inner calm that meditation can unfold.

The practice of meditation triggers the body's relaxation response, resulting in a reduction in stress hormone levels, such as cortisol. Mindfulness practices impart the ability to respond to stressors with composure, diminishing the overall perception of stress. Consistent meditation is linked to alterations in the amygdala, a region of the brain, fostering improved emotional regulation. This enhancement in emotional management contributes to a greater capacity to navigate and manage emotions, ultimately mitigating the impact of emotional challenges.

Meditation yields heightened focus and attention, coupled with physical benefits such as neuroplasticity changes in the brain, particularly in regions linked to attention and concentration. This translates into an improved capacity to sustain attention and focus, both during meditation and in daily activities. Additionally, there is a decrease in amygdala activation associated with the brain's fear response.

Mindfulness-based interventions have demonstrated efficacy in alleviating symptoms of anxiety disorders and fostering a sense of calm. Furthermore, meditation induces a state of relaxation, resulting in reduced blood pressure and a lowered risk of cardiovascular events. This contributes significantly to overall heart health.

Meditation exerts a positive influence on the production of sleep-inducing hormones, notably melatonin. This enhancement in sleep patterns and the overall quality of sleep contributes to heightened mental health and improved well-being. Mindfulness meditation brings about alterations in pain perception and diminishes the activation of brain regions linked to pain. This results in an improvement in pain tolerance and coping mechanisms, positioning meditation as a valuable complementary approach in pain management.

Furthermore, meditation is associated with enhanced immune function, potentially attributed to stress reduction and overall improvements in health. This underscores its broader impact on promoting overall well-being and resilience.

Meditation diminishes susceptibility to illness and facilitates swifter recovery times. It instigates beneficial changes in the brain, augmenting cognitive function and fortifying resilience against age-related cognitive decline.

Mindfulness-based interventions prove effective in mitigating symptoms of depression and preventing relapse. This practice augments connectivity between brain regions linked to self-awareness and introspection, ultimately refining the understanding of one's thoughts and emotions, thereby fostering emotional intelligence.

Meditation fosters robust connections between mental and physical well-being by elevating awareness of the intricate connection between thoughts, emotions, and bodily sensations. This practice initiates positive changes in brain regions linked to empathy and social connection, resulting in heightened interpersonal skills, empathy, and communication. These improvements contribute to enhanced relationships and overall health outcomes, encompassing cardiovascular health, immune function, and longevity.

The exploration of the physical and mental health benefits of mindfulness and meditation underscores the holistic impact these practices can have on individuals, promoting both physical resilience and mental well-being. Incorporating mindfulness into daily life emerges as a potent approach for cultivating a healthy and balanced mind-body connection.

Mindfulness and meditation techniques frequently initiate the body's relaxation response, activating the parasympathetic nervous system. This physiological shift acts as a counterforce to the stress response, fostering a state of calmness.

Given that chronic stress is linked to heightened cortisol levels, mindfulness practices play a role in regulating cortisol production, thereby mitigating the impact of stress on the body by cultivating non-judgmental awareness of thoughts, feelings, and external stimuli. By mindfully acknowledging stressors, individuals can approach them with curiosity and openness, diminishing the automatic and reactive stress response.

Mindfulness fosters a non-reactive and non-judgmental awareness of emotions, diminishing emotional reactivity to stressors. This equips individuals with the capacity to respond with heightened composure and resilience. The practice of mindfulness further promotes the cultivation of healthier coping mechanisms. Instead of impulsively reacting to stress, individuals learn to respond mindfully, opting for actions that align with their values and contribute to their long-term well-being.

By nurturing a robust mind-body connection, individuals can identify and address physical manifestations of stress, such as muscle tension or shallow breathing. This integrated approach facilitates a more integrated strategy for stress reduction. Mindfulness encourages individuals to approach stressors with a mindset centred on acceptance and non-resistance. This mindset, in turn, nurtures the development of coping strategies that are mindful, adaptive, and less likely to contribute to additional stress.

Mindfulness plays a pivotal role in the development of psychological resilience, equipping individuals to rebound more effectively from stressful situations. This resilience is nurtured through the cultivation of a present-moment awareness that enables individuals to navigate challenges with a balanced perspective.

Mindfulness promotes an acceptance of uncertainty and impermanence. By approaching uncertainties with mindful awareness, individuals can alleviate anxiety and stress associated with the unknown, redirecting their focus to the present moment.

Partake in mindful savouring of positive moments, whether it's relishing a sunset, enjoying a cup of tea, or engaging in a pleasant conversation. Take a moment to wholeheartedly appreciate the richness of the experience. Cultivate gratitude by reflecting on things you're thankful for each day.

By training the mind to stay present, mindfulness aids in reducing distractions and resisting the allure of unrelated thoughts. The practice of mindfulness fosters an elevated awareness of the present moment, enhancing the ability to discern and appreciate details in one's surroundings.

This heightened diligence contributes to improvements in decision-making and problem-solving skills. It imparts the skill of gently redirecting attention to the present moment when the mind begins to wander. This reduction in mind-wandering not only enhances cognitive efficiency but also serves as a safeguard against the mental fatigue associated with constant distraction.

Mindfulness practices, exemplified by open awareness meditation, nurture cognitive flexibility, the adeptness to adapt and seamlessly transition between various cognitive tasks or perspectives. This flexibility proves advantageous for effective problem-solving and smoothly adjusting to changing circumstances.

The influence of mindfulness extends positively to memory function, particularly in areas such as working memory and the capacity to retain and recall information. Practices like mindfulness-based stress reduction (MBSR) have demonstrated notable positive effects on memory.

Mindfulness practices play a pivotal role in regulating emotions, serving as a preventive measure against emotional hijacking that could otherwise impede cognitive functioning. The regulation of emotions contributes to a stable and focused mind, laying the foundation for optimal cognitive performance.

Mindfulness, with its emphasis on a non-judgmental and open-minded approach to challenges, fosters a mindset that enhances critical thinking skills. This approach promotes creative thinking and encourages the exploration of various solutions.

Mindfulness is linked to enhancements in executive functions, encompassing cognitive processes like planning, organising, and decision-making. The bolstering of executive function plays a pivotal role in facilitating effective goal setting and execution. Research indicates that mindfulness practices may exert a decelerating effect on age-related cognitive decline.

Consistent engagement in meditation is correlated with positive changes in brain structure and function, thereby contributing to cognitive resilience among older adults. Furthermore, mindfulness practices serve to clear mental clutter and foster mental clarity. This heightened mental clarity enables individuals to approach tasks with a focused and unclouded mind.

Mindfulness elevates awareness of problems and challenges without inducing overwhelm. This heightened problem awareness paves the way for a more strategic and mindful approach to addressing issues. The practice of mindfulness and meditation plays a role in managing mental fatigue by fostering relaxation and preventing cognitive overload.

This, in turn, contributes to sustained cognitive performance throughout the day. Mindfulness practices also stimulate divergent thinking and creativity. By nurturing an open and receptive mindset, individuals are more likely to generate creative ideas and innovative solutions.

Mindfulness serves as a valuable tool in regulating negative emotions like anger, anxiety, or sadness. By consciously acknowledging and accepting these emotions without judgment, individuals can prevent their escalation and interference with overall well-being. Central to mindfulness is the emphasis on accepting all emotions, even the challenging ones. Rather than suppressing or avoiding difficult emotions, individuals learn to acknowledge and accept them, fostering emotional resilience.

Mindfulness practices extend their focus to cultivating positive emotions, including gratitude, compassion, and joy. Striking a balance between acknowledging and transforming negative emotions, while nurturing positive emotions plays a crucial role in fostering emotional well-being and resilience.

The practice of mindfulness encourages an acceptance of uncertainty and impermanence, equipping individuals with the skills to navigate emotionally challenging situations. This enables them to maintain balance and composure even in the face of uncertainty. Mindfulness practices also permeate interpersonal interactions, enhancing emotional regulation in relationships. By infusing mindfulness into communication, individuals can respond to others with empathy, active listening, and emotional intelligence.

Let go of expectations and perfectionism. Mindfulness centres around the journey rather than reaching a predefined outcome. Direct your attention to the process rather than fixating on the results. Take time to acknowledge and celebrate small successes and progress along the way. Divide your practice into easily digestible segments and recognise resistance as a natural part of the process.

Understand that change is a gradual process, so initiate your mindfulness journey with practices that align with your current comfort level. Introduce new elements gradually as you become more familiar and comfortable with the practice.

Mindfulness-based interventions prove effective in transforming the perception of pain. By altering the mind's response to pain signals, individuals can find relief from both chronic and acute pain. This reduction in pain perception not only contributes to enhanced mental well-being but also facilitates better physical functioning. Furthermore, mindfulness practices play a role in promoting relaxation, fostering an environment conducive to improved sleep.

Chronic inflammation is linked to an array of physical and mental health conditions. Mindfulness practices are thought to exert anti-inflammatory effects, thereby contributing to improved overall health. The reduction in inflammation levels can have a positive impact on conditions such as arthritis, cardiovascular disease, and mental health disorders.

The emphasis on present-moment awareness in mindfulness cultivates a robust mind-body connection. Elevated body awareness enables individuals to identify and address physical sensations associated with stress or tension, ultimately promoting comprehensive well-being.

Emerging research indicates that mindfulness practices might have an impact on the gut-brain axis, influencing digestive health. A healthy gut plays a pivotal role in overall well-being, exerting effects on both mental and physical health. Engaging in mindfulness practices, particularly activities like yoga, has the potential to enhance physical performance. This improvement in physical performance contributes to comprehensive physical health and well-being, exerting positive influences on mood and cognitive function.

Mindfulness and meditation serve as catalysts for regular self-reflection, creating valuable opportunities to delve into personal beliefs, values, and aspirations. Through this process of self-reflection, individuals gain insights into their motivations, desires, and areas for personal growth, contributing to a more authentic and aligned sense of self.

Being fully present in each moment enables individuals to engage more authentically with themselves and others, fostering a profound sense of presence and connection in daily life. Mindfulness entails observing habitual thought patterns and behaviours without attachment. The heightened self-awareness cultivated through mindfulness allows individuals to identify and understand automatic habits, marking a crucial step in breaking free from unhelpful patterns and fostering positive change.

Mindfulness practices play a pivotal role in aiding individuals to discern their values and life purpose through deliberate exploration. Armed with a clearer sense of purpose, individuals can align their actions with their values, thereby contributing to a life that is more meaningful and fulfilling.

Central to mindfulness is the emphasis on self-compassion and the acceptance of oneself, which includes recognising imperfections and vulnerabilities. Through the practice of self-compassion, individuals cultivate a kinder and more understanding relationship with themselves, fostering resilience and nurturing a positive self-image.

Mindfulness seamlessly integrates into interpersonal communication, championing active listening and considerate expression. Through the cultivation of mindful communication, individuals elevate their capacity to convey thoughts authentically and empathetically, thereby fostering deeper connections with others.

Mindfulness practices encompass an expansion of awareness beyond subjective experiences to embrace broader perspectives. This widening of awareness nurtures a profound sense of interconnectedness and empathy, thereby contributing to personal growth by expanding one's understanding of the world and fostering a compassionate outlook.

Mindfulness inspires individuals to engage with experiences patiently, embracing the unfolding of each moment. The cultivation of patience becomes a catalyst for personal growth, diminishing impulsivity, fostering thoughtful decision-making, and enhancing resilience in the face of challenges. Mindfulness meditation, a key practice, entails training the mind to maintain focus on a chosen point of attention, such as the breath. This intentional focus serves as a cornerstone in the development of patience and the broader benefits it bestows.

Enhanced concentration and focus serve as catalysts for improved cognitive abilities, empowering individuals to immerse themselves more completely in tasks and activities and thereby fostering personal and professional growth. Mindfulness, as a practice, prompts individuals to scrutinise and question limiting beliefs without judgment. The acknowledgment and release of self-limiting beliefs pave the way for new possibilities, nurturing personal growth and a profound sense of empowerment.

Evaluating the impact of mindfulness and meditation on one's life is a contemplative and introspective endeavour. While the benefits of these practices may be subjective, there are several methods individuals can employ to assess their impact.

Maintaining a journal to regularly record experiences with mindfulness and meditation is one effective approach. This involves noting thoughts, emotions, and any observed changes in daily life. Consistently tracking this journey over time provides valuable insights into patterns, progress, and areas for further exploration.

Precisely articulate your intentions and objectives for engaging in mindfulness and meditation. Consistently revisit and evaluate whether your actions align with these intentions. Establishing clear goals serves as a structured basis for assessment, enabling you to measure the tangible changes you aspire to make.

Incorporate well-being scales or assessments that quantify experiences into your routine. These may encompass scales gauging stress, anxiety, depression, and overall life satisfaction. Regularly undertaking these assessments facilitates tracking changes in well-being and identifying areas that may warrant further attention.

Evaluate your comprehensive quality of life, considering physical, mental, and social well-being. Utilise established and validated scales designed to measure different facets of life quality. Monitoring alterations in your overall quality of life offers a holistic perspective on how mindfulness and meditation influence various dimensions of your well-being.

Pay close attention to your daily behaviours, reactions, and responses. Observe any changes in how you navigate challenges, engage with others, or manage stress. Positive shifts in behaviour, such as heightened patience, improved communication, or the adoption of healthier habits, may serve as indicators of the impact of mindfulness and meditation.

Create detailed action plans grounded in mindfulness principles, such as integrating mindful eating or mindful breathing exercises into daily routines. Assess your commitment to these action plans to gauge the effective integration of mindfulness into your daily life. Monitor physiological indicators like heart rate, blood pressure, or cortisol levels before and after engaging in mindfulness or meditation. Shifts in these markers can signify the calming and stress-reducing impact of these practices.

Evaluate cognitive functions such as attention, memory, and executive function, as mindfulness has been linked to improvements in these areas. Recognising enhancements in cognitive function serves as evidence of the cognitive benefits derived from mindfulness and meditation.

Reflect on your responses to stress or challenging situations and evaluate whether mindfulness techniques are naturally incorporated during these moments. The spontaneous application of mindfulness in real-life situations indicates the practical impact of these practices on stress management.

Examine changes in your relationships and observe whether you engage in interactions with enhanced empathy, active listening, or improved communication. Positive shifts in relationship dynamics serve as indicators of the social benefits derived from mindfulness and meditation.

If you're enrolled in a structured mindfulness program, such as MBSR, share your feedback on your experiences. Evaluate program components, the effectiveness of facilitators, and your own level of engagement. Conduct periodic self-assessments, whether monthly or quarterly, to reflect on your overall well-being, challenges, and successes. Long-term reflection provides a comprehensive view of the cumulative impact of mindfulness and meditation on your life.

Engage in discussions about your experiences with mindfulness and meditation with qualified instructors or mental health professionals. Seeking professional guidance offers personalised insights and recommendations tailored to your unique journey.

Connect with others who practise mindfulness, sharing experiences and participating in group discussions to cultivate a sense of shared growth. Utilise tracking features on mindfulness apps to monitor your usage, progress, and self-reported changes in well-being. App data can serve as a quantitative measure of your engagement and consistency in mindfulness practices.

Evaluating the influence of mindfulness and meditation encompasses a multifaceted approach, blending self-reflection, behavioural observation, and well-being assessments. A commitment to consistent and sincere self-assessment, coupled with openness to adaptation and exploration, empowers individuals to glean valuable insights into the transformative effects of these practices on their lives. It's crucial to recognise that the impact of mindfulness and meditation is often subtle and cumulative, necessitating ongoing attention and self-awareness.

Chapter 9 - Cultivating Healthy Relationships and Social Connections

Cultivating healthy relationships and nurturing meaningful social connections stand as fundamental pillars in the tapestry of human existence, exerting a profound influence across diverse facets of our lives. Beyond the immediate emotional fulfilment, robust social bonds have been intricately linked to a plethora of health benefits, encompassing both mental and physical well-being.

As we navigate the intricate web of relationships, ranging from family and friendships to romantic partnerships and professional connections, the dynamics, qualities, and communication skills involved play a pivotal role in determining the overall health and vitality of these connections. Recognising the significance of healthy relationships and social connections for overall well-being is crucial for understanding how human connections profoundly impact various aspects of an individual's life.

The role of social connections in mental health is pivotal, it contributes to diminished stress levels and heightened emotional resilience. Positive relationships offer crucial emotional support, decreasing the likelihood of mental health issues such as depression and anxiety. There is a strong correlation between robust social connections and extended life expectancy. Those with fulfilling relationships typically enjoy longer, healthier lives, with such connections acting as a buffer against stress and aiding individuals in coping with life's challenges.

Emotional support from friends, family, and loved ones can mitigate the impact of stressful situations. Relationships contribute to a sense of belonging and identity, fostering a positive self-image. Feeling connected to a community or social group provides a support system that enhances overall well-being. Healthy relationships offer a safe space for emotional expression and regulation. Interpersonal connections can assist in processing emotions and finding constructive ways to manage them.

Profound connections hold a significant sway over one's joy and contentment in life. The synergy of shared moments, laughter, and companionship intricately composes a tapestry of positivity in our outlook. Engaging socially and partaking in enriching conversations not only fosters cognitive advantages but also acts as a bulwark against the perils of cognitive decline. Intellectual nourishment within relationships ensures the mind's vigour, potentially mitigating the risk of mental deterioration.

In the realm of well-being, robust relationships become the fertile soil for personal evolution and the unearthing of self. A supportive network not only propels individuals towards their aspirations but also emboldens them to embrace risks and delve into uncharted facets of their being.

In times of adversity, social bonds emerge as a valuable asset, cultivating resilience. The awareness of a supportive network empowers individuals, enhancing their ability to adeptly navigate challenging circumstances. Favourable connections within the professional realm not only contribute to a more robust and productive work environment but also plays a pivotal role in diminishing workplace stress and elevating job satisfaction. Engaging in social and community endeavours serves to fortify these connections, fostering a sense of shared purpose and bolstering societal well-being.

The calibre of parent-child relationships holds substantial sway over a child's emotional and psychological maturation. Secure attachments forged in childhood complexly shape the bedrock of future well-being. The emphasis here lies not merely in the quantity of relationships but rather in the substance of those connections.

Profound and meaningful bonds frequently exert a deeper influence on well-being than numerous superficial ties. The advent of technology has undoubtedly altered the terrain of social connections. While digital bonds can be valuable, the richness of face-to-face interactions often proves more advantageous for overall well-being.

Significant connections are tied to heightened positive emotions, playing a pivotal role in elevating one's overall mood. The act of celebrating successes and sharing moments of joy with others becomes a catalyst for enhancing emotional well-being. Positive relationships demonstrate a correlation with a fortified immune system, diminishing susceptibility to illnesses.

The provision of social support is notably associated with lower blood pressure, fostering cardiovascular health. Notably, robust social connections have been identified as a key factor in an extended life expectancy and improved overall physical well-being. In the face of stress, positive relationships emerge as a protective shield, mitigating the detrimental effects and promoting resilience to stressors.

Robust relationships form the bedrock for adept conflict resolution, fostering a constructive approach. Supportive connections function as catalysts, motivating individuals to chase after personal goals and aspirations. The realm of positive relationships becomes a fertile ground for feedback and introspective moments, nurturing individual growth. Mental resilience, a key asset in facing life's trials, is nurtured within positive relationships. The complex embroidery of mental health is woven closely with the quality of social connections and relationships.

Exploring diverse relationship types offers a nuanced understanding of the manifold dynamics, expectations, and influences embedded in human connections. Familial relationships, frequently serving as the bedrock of an individual's support system, are distinguished by unconditional love and acceptance.

The existence of defined roles and expectations within families nurtures a profound sense of belonging. Friendships, on the other hand, emerge as voluntary alliances grounded in shared interests and values. Friends play pivotal roles in offering emotional support, understanding, and companionship, spanning the spectrum from casual acquaintances to enduring, lifelong bonds.

Romantic relationships entail a profound connection marked by both emotional and physical intimacy. The bedrock of healthy romantic partnerships lies in effective communication and the cultivation of trust. These relationships encompass the joint navigation of challenges, fostering mutual growth. Professional relationships, alternatively, are often constructed upon the pillars of collaboration, teamwork, and shared objectives. Mentoring relationships play pivotal roles in fostering professional development and personal growth.

Parents assume the role of influential role models, shaping a child's values and behaviours. As children transition into adulthood, the dynamics of parent-child relationships undergo a natural evolution. Sibling relationships, marked by a blend of camaraderie and occasional conflicts, carve out their own unique space. Connections with extended family members contribute to a broader sense of community and shared history, often playing a pivotal role in passing down cultural traditions.

Long-term couples, in the journey of their relationship, encounter growth, commitment, and a tapestry of shared life experiences. The success of these enduring bonds lies in the adept navigation of life changes and challenges. A delicate balance is maintained between preserving individual identities and fostering a shared life. Casual relationships on the other hand involve minimal commitment and may be of short-term duration.

Casual relationships, whether recreational, social, or rooted in shared interests, thrive on clear communication of expectations. Online relationships, fostered through digital platforms and social media, necessitate overcoming challenges such as miscommunication to become meaningful connections. Platonic friendships, marked by deep connections without romantic entanglement, are characterised by emotional intimacy and shared experiences.

A considerable number of these platonic friendships endure a lifetime, providing lasting and unwavering support. In-law relationships entail the blending of diverse family structures and dynamics. The establishment of clear boundaries emerges as a crucial factor in fostering healthy connections with in-laws. Positive in-law relationships, in turn, extend and enrich broader support systems within the family.

Transparent and candid communication is imperative in fostering healthy relationships. Within families, expressing feelings and concerns openly proves beneficial, while establishing and honouring boundaries promotes mutual respect and understanding. The fabric of familial bonds is reinforced through the quality time spent together, giving rise to lasting memories from shared experiences.

In the realm of friendships, trust serves as the foundational pillar. Trust is cultivated over time through reliability and loyalty. Healthy friendships, marked by mutual support and a reciprocal give-and-take, thrive on balanced efforts from both parties. Embracing each other's flaws and differences stands as a pivotal aspect of genuine friendship.

At the heart of comprehending each other's needs and viewpoints rests the bedrock of effective communication, a realm that embraces the art of active listening. Within the realm of romantic entanglements, a deep connection flourishes through the channels of emotional intimacy and shared vulnerability. Couples, who seamlessly unite as a cohesive team, especially in the face of adversities, invariably sow the seeds of robust and flourishing relationships.

Turning our gaze toward the professional sphere, positive work relationships find their roots in collaborative efforts and a collective dedication to the pursuit of shared objectives. The cultivation of a thriving workplace dynamic necessitates the artful interplay of constructive feedback and the acknowledgment of accomplishments. Moreover, the mitigation of misunderstandings is aptly facilitated by the meticulous establishment of transparent expectations.

Cultivating a nurturing atmosphere where children feel both heard and valued is pivotal for fostering a healthy parent-child relationship. Striking a delicate balance between providing guidance and allowing space for independence is crucial for a child's growth. The parent-child bond is fortified through spending quality time engaging in various activities together.

In the realm of sibling relationships, the application of effective conflict resolution and communication skills proves beneficial. Strengthening connections with extended family members is achieved through engaging in shared family traditions. Furthermore, promoting harmony within the family involves embracing differences and celebrating the unique personalities within the familial unit

Couples who share long-term goals and aspirations often find themselves in healthier relationships. Relationship longevity is bolstered when partners demonstrate adaptability to life changes and evolve together. Essential for the sustenance of a healthy long-term relationship is the practice of respectful communication, even during disagreements.

Clear communication of expectations proves pivotal in preventing misunderstandings within casual relationships. In the context of casual connections, a positive dynamic is fostered through engaging in enjoyable activities together. Respecting each other's boundaries remains crucial for mutual respect, even in casual relationships. For online relationships to thrive, effective digital communication and an understanding of the limitations inherent in virtual interactions are key components.

Discovering shared interests online serves as a foundation for cultivating meaningful connections. Maintaining a balance between online and offline interactions proves crucial for the vitality of virtual relationships. Fostering emotional intimacy within platonic friendships is achieved through engaging in deep and meaningful conversations. The strength of platonic friendships is further fortified by demonstrating reliability and being a source of support during times of need.

The bedrock of robust relationships lies in effective communication, cultivating understanding, trust, and connection. Openness is the lifeblood of healthy relationships, and it thrives on transparent communication about thoughts, feelings, and concerns. Trust is solidified through honesty, establishing a foundation for a robust and resilient connection.

Actively engaging in attentive listening to your partner, family member, or friend is crucial. Demonstrate genuine interest and involvement in what they share. Listening with empathy goes beyond words, understanding the emotions beneath the surface, and it serves as a catalyst for fostering a profound and meaningful connection.

Articulate your needs and expectations with clarity, as ambiguity can breed misunderstanding and frustration. Healthy communication necessitates negotiation and the discovery of common ground to satisfy each other's needs. When delivering feedback, centre your focus on the positive aspects.

Constructive feedback, emphasising growth rather than criticism, is key. Specify behaviours or situations, avoiding generalisations, as this clarity aids in understanding and improvement. Tackle conflicts promptly to prevent the accumulation of resentment. Timely communication is the path to effective resolution.

Employ "I" statements when expressing feelings to avoid placing blame on the other person, fostering a less defensive response. Be attentive to non-verbal cues, such as body language and facial expressions, as they often convey emotions that words may not capture. Sustain eye contact to convey both attentiveness and sincerity, establishing a connection and signalling active listening. Set and respect boundaries regarding when and where to broach specific topics to ensure a comfortable environment for all involved.

Acknowledge and honour each other's preferred communication styles, recognising that some may lean towards directness, while others may prefer a more subtle approach. Provide verbal affirmations and encouragement, as positive communication is instrumental in fostering a supportive and uplifting atmosphere.

Reinforce positive behaviour by expressing gratitude and appreciation, thereby strengthening the bond. Acknowledge and respect cultural differences in communication styles, fostering cultural sensitivity that promotes understanding and prevents misunderstandings.

Acquire proficient cross-cultural communication skills to navigate diverse relationships successfully. Ensure clarity in written communication to avoid misinterpretation, as tone can be easily misunderstood in digital messages. Strike a balance between digital and face-to-face communication, as the latter often provides more contextual understanding.

In intimate relationships, healthy communication entails expressing vulnerabilities without the fear of judgment. Find equilibrium between autonomy and togetherness, and effective communication becomes instrumental in navigating these dynamic interactions.

Mindful communication necessitates being fully present in the conversation, avoiding distractions, and directing focus towards the speaker. Listening without judgment is key in fostering acceptance and understanding. In relationships encountering challenges, couples can benefit from seeking counselling as it provides a neutral space for improving communication.

Attending workshops on conflict resolution aids in acquiring practical skills for handling disagreements constructively. Effective communication is an ongoing process demanding effort, understanding, and adaptability. When cultivated as a skill, it becomes the foundation of healthy relationships, fostering intimacy, trust, and mutual growth.

Active listening is a foundational communication skill encompassing full concentration, understanding, responsive engagement, and retention of communicated information. It elevates the quality of interpersonal relationships and is instrumental in achieving effective communication.

The key components of active listening include nonverbal cues, such as demonstrating engagement through eye contact, nodding, and open body language. Verbal affirmations involve using cues like "I see," "I understand," or paraphrasing to convey attentiveness.

Avoid interruptions by allowing the speaker to express themselves fully before responding. Active listening is the linchpin for gaining a profound understanding of the speaker's perspective and plays a pivotal role in conflict resolution by ensuring everyone feels heard.

Experiencing active listening fosters a sense of trust and rapport in relationships. Sidestep distractions, offering your undivided attention to the speaker. Clarify points when needed and summarise key messages to confirm understanding. Demonstrate empathy by acknowledging the speaker's feelings and emotions.

Assertiveness entails the capacity to openly and honestly express thoughts, feelings, and needs while concurrently respecting the rights and opinions of others. This vital communication skill is essential for establishing healthy boundaries and upholding self-respect.

Assertive individuals adeptly articulate their needs and preferences without resorting to passivity or aggression. Assertiveness involves communicating with clarity while still honouring the rights and opinions of others. Typically, assertive communication is accompanied by confident and positive body language.

Embracing assertiveness contributes significantly to cultivating a positive self-image and boosting self-esteem. This skill proves invaluable in addressing conflicts directly and seeking constructive solutions. In the realm of relationships, assertiveness plays a pivotal role by fostering open and honest communication, thereby nurturing the health of the relationship.

Learning to assertively say "no" is essential for establishing and maintaining boundaries. When expressing feelings and needs, utilising "I" statements helps avoid sounding accusatory. It is crucial to maintain a firm yet respectful stance when articulating thoughts or boundaries.

Empathy entails comprehending and sharing the feelings of another person, serving as a crucial element of effective communication that enhances emotional intelligence and facilitates relationship-building. It involves grasping the perspective and emotions of others and actively participating in their emotional experiences. Taking appropriate action to offer support and comfort exemplifies empathetic behaviour.

In relationships, empathy fosters a profound sense of connection and mutual understanding, playing a pivotal role in conflict resolution by validating the feelings of all parties involved. Empathetic communication becomes a cornerstone in building trust and rapport by sincerely acknowledging and respecting the emotions of others.

Engage in active listening, demonstrating sincere interest in the experiences and feelings shared by others. Acknowledge and validate the emotions expressed by those around you. Practice suspending judgment and strive to understand situations from the perspective of the other person. By combining active listening, assertiveness, and empathy, a potent synergy is formed in communication.

Recognise the appropriateness of each skill and adapt communication based on the context and relationship. Active listening, assertiveness, and empathy are interconnected abilities that play a role in effective and respectful communication. Proficiency in these skills elevates interpersonal relationships, nurtures understanding, and cultivates a positive communication environment.

Trust serves as a cornerstone in all healthy relationships, be it within family, friendship, romantic partnerships, or professional connections. Grasping the significance of trust and employing strategies to construct and preserve it proves essential in nurturing robust and enduring relationships.

Trust involves relying on the integrity, strength, ability, or surety of an individual or entity, embodying a belief in their reliability, truthfulness, or capability. It establishes the foundation for mutual understanding and cooperation, demanding consistency and dependability in both words and actions. Honesty, transparency, and moral character are pivotal components of integrity, further bolstering the framework of trust in any relationship.

Comprehend and consider the feelings and perspectives of others. The establishment of trust is fortified through open and honest communication. Consistency arises from predictability and stability over time. Trust, serving as the cornerstone, is paramount in the construction and sustenance of healthy relationships. It cultivates a profound sense of emotional safety and security. Furthermore, trust acts as a catalyst, fostering collaboration, cooperation, and the facilitation of effective teamwork.

Cultivate trust through the practice of open and honest communication, emphasising the avoidance of deception. Actively listen to others, displaying that you genuinely value their perspectives. Bolster trust by unwaveringly following through on promises and commitments, thereby fostering reliability.

Enhance trust by infusing predictability into your behaviour. Even in challenging situations, prioritise truthfulness, recognising that honesty forms the bedrock of trust. Display understanding and empathy towards the feelings and experiences of others as part of the trust-building process.

Recognise and validate the emotions expressed by others, cultivating an emotional connection. Demonstrate consideration and respect for the autonomy of others by respecting personal boundaries. To prevent misunderstandings, clearly communicate expectations.

Acknowledge and take responsibility for mistakes, offering sincere apologies when necessary to convey a commitment to repairing trust. Establish trust through sustained reliability over an extended period. Demonstrate a dedication to personal growth and improvement in the trust-building process.

Address conflicts in a constructive manner, focusing on understanding and resolution rather than assigning blame. Incorporate the practices of apologising and forgiving into the process of restoring trust. Strengthen the bond between individuals by creating positive memories and sharing experiences.

Celebrate achievements and successes together to fortify the connection. Foster an understanding and respect for diverse perspectives and cultural differences. Be attuned to the cultural context in which trust is developed and maintained.

Preventing disappointment and nurturing trust involves setting realistic expectations that align with reality. Breaches of trust can result from a failure to establish and respect personal boundaries. Trust is an ongoing process demanding commitment, communication, and mutual respect for the enduring well-being of any relationship.

Examining the elements that lead to the deterioration of trust and uncovering effective strategies to restore it is a vital component of sustaining healthy relationships. Deceptive behaviour, encompassing actions like lying or withholding information, has the potential to significantly undermine trust in a relationship.

Whether in minor or substantial matters, repetitive betrayals contribute to a gradual erosion of trust over time. A deficiency in open, transparent, and honest communication nurtures misunderstandings, ultimately leading to a breakdown in trust.

Disregarding or violating personal boundaries erodes the sense of safety and trust within a relationship. A consistent failure to fulfil promises and commitments diminishes trust in one's reliability. Ignoring or mishandling conflicts without resolution can foster resentment and further erode the foundation of trust.

Recognise the impact of actions that contribute to the erosion of trust. Extend a genuine and sincere apology, demonstrating remorse for the breach of trust. Promote open dialogue to comprehend each other's perspectives and feelings.

Cultivate an atmosphere of honesty and openness as a foundation for rebuilding trust. Set clear expectations for behaviour and commitments to mitigate future misunderstandings. Demonstrate unwavering consistency and reliability in actions, aligning behaviour with commitments.

Recognise that rebuilding trust is a gradual process demanding sustained effort. Display a commitment to respecting and honouring personal boundaries. Foster discussions about boundaries to proactively prevent future breaches. Consider engaging the assistance of counsellors or mediators to facilitate constructive conversations and resolutions.

Evident changes in behaviour should be displayed gradually to rebuild trust. Consistently display positive and trustworthy actions over an extended period. Promote self-reflection and learning from mistakes to prevent recurrence.

Exhibit a commitment to personal growth and improvement. Forge new positive memories and shared experiences to reconstruct the emotional connection. Acknowledge and celebrate milestones and positive changes within the relationship. Collaborate to establish shared goals, nurturing a sense of unity and purpose.

Conflict is an inherent and unavoidable aspect of any relationship. Yet, the way conflicts are addressed and resolved significantly impacts the overall health and durability of the relationship. Acknowledging the inevitability of conflicts and embracing healthy resolution strategies is crucial for sustaining robust and resilient connections. Recognise conflicts as a natural facet of any relationship, stemming from differences in perspectives, values, and expectations.

Consider conflicts as opportunities for growth, understanding, and fortifying the relationship through effective resolution. Misunderstandings, poor communication, or a lack of clarity can often be precursors to conflicts. Conflicts often arise from unfulfilled expectations or mismatched assumptions about roles and responsibilities. Differences in core values and beliefs can also lead to conflicts, especially when making important life decisions. External pressures, such as work-related stress or financial challenges, may further contribute to conflicts.

Cultivate an environment of open and active listening to comprehend each other's perspectives. Encourage the constructive expression of feelings and thoughts. Maintain focus on the specific issue at hand rather than resorting to blame. Use respectful language and tone to foster a positive atmosphere. Strive to understand the other person's point of view with empathy. Validate each other's feelings to create a sense of understanding.

Clearly communicate individual boundaries to avoid future conflicts. Cultivate a culture of respecting each other's personal space and limits. Approach conflicts as a team, working together to find mutually beneficial solutions. Engage in collaborative brainstorming to explore multiple solutions. If emotions run high, take a break to cool down before continuing the conversation. Use the break to reflect on personal feelings and perspectives.

Maintain a laser-like focus on the present challenge, avoiding the rehashing of historical conflicts. Redirect the dialogue towards constructive solutions, steering clear of prolonged discussions on past issues. Enlist the aid of an impartial third party to mediate conversations and provide valuable guidance. Embrace a mindset of growth when confronted with conflicts, acknowledging them as chances for both personal and relational development.

Persistently glean insights from conflicts to enhance communication and comprehension. Extend genuine apologies when warranted, assuming accountability for one's actions. Foster a mindset of forgiveness to liberate oneself from resentment and forge ahead. All parties involved should articulate a dedication to resolving conflicts in a constructive manner. Recognise that achieving resolution is an ongoing journey, demanding a commitment to long-term relational well-being.

Boundaries delineate the parameters of acceptable behaviour, creating an environment where individuals experience a sense of safety, respect, and understanding. These boundaries encompass physical, emotional, and mental limits that individuals set to safeguard their well-being and preserve a sense of autonomy. The establishment of boundaries empowers individuals to uphold their autonomy, safeguarding their self-identity and personal space.

Well-defined boundaries play a crucial role in fostering healthy, harmonious, and respectful relationships. The act of setting boundaries empowers individuals to articulate their needs and preferences, nurturing a profound sense of control. Within families, the establishment of clear boundaries ensures the preservation of each member's autonomy while sustaining an intense sense of familial connection. Similarly, in friendships, boundaries serve to navigate expectations, forestall misunderstandings, and cultivate a foundation of mutual respect.

Establishing boundaries in romantic relationships is vital for preserving individual identities, nurturing intimacy, and securing emotional safety. In the workplace, boundaries contribute to a favourable environment for collaboration, effective communication, and professional development. The fear of conflict or rejection can pose challenges in communicating and setting boundaries for individuals. Additionally, societal norms and cultural influences may impact an individual's capacity to effectively establish and communicate boundaries.

Reacting assertively to breaches of boundaries entails articulating discomfort or disagreement while upholding respect. Managing such violations through conflict resolution not only promotes understanding but also fortifies relationships. In the workplace, setting boundaries is instrumental in maintaining a healthy work-life balance, thwarting burnout, and alleviating stress. Professional boundaries among colleagues guarantee mutual respect, contributing to a positive and collaborative work atmosphere.

Honouring boundaries is an acknowledgment and safeguarding of personal integrity, fostering an atmosphere of mutual respect. Transparent boundaries offer individuals space to openly communicate their needs, preferences, and expectations. Robustly defined boundaries diminish the chances of misunderstanding by clearly articulating and agreeing upon expectations.

Emotional safety is cultivated through boundaries, signifying the recognition, value, and protection of feelings. Upholding emotional boundaries prevents emotional exhaustion and guarantees that individuals feel secure in expressing their emotions.

Precisely outlined physical boundaries, encompass aspects like personal space and privacy, it plays a pivotal role in fostering feelings of respect and understanding. Emotional boundaries function as guardians of personal space, delineating emotional independence and avoiding emotional entanglement.

Clearly conveyed boundaries serve as a proactive measure, mitigating the risk of conflicts escalating to detrimental levels. Established boundaries serve as a structured framework for resolving conflicts with respect, guiding discussions and the formulation of solutions.

Upholding boundaries cultivates empathy by nurturing an appreciation for others' perspectives and needs. Boundaries pave the way for compassionate responses as individuals navigate each other's emotional landscapes with sensitivity. Well-defined boundaries empower individuals to advocate for their needs and stand resolute in their values. The soil for mutual respect becomes fertile when individuals feel empowered to assert their boundaries in a manner that is both respectful and considerate.

Boundaries instil predictability and consistency, fostering a sense of trust and reliability in relationships. Demonstrating steadfast respect for boundaries consistently underscores reliability and strengthens trust within the relationship. Recognising and honouring cultural differences in boundary-setting enhances mutual respect and appreciation. Flexibility in boundary respect, contextually applied, ensures a nuanced and adaptable approach to fostering mutual understanding.

Well-nurtured connections serve as a sturdy emotional support system, bolstering resilience in the face of challenges. Diversifying social connections in terms of quantity provides exposure to a range of perspectives and experiences, ultimately enriching one's life. Maintaining enough social connections is crucial in warding off social isolation, a factor associated with various mental and physical health issues.

Achieving equilibrium between profound, meaningful connections and a broad social network ensures the cultivation of a holistic and supportive social environment. Striking a balance between both quality and quantity enables individuals to tailor their social support to diverse needs and circumstances.

Connections imbued with emotional resonance have a positive influence on mental well-being, cultivating feelings of belonging and acceptance. A diverse array of social connections contributes to mental well-being by mitigating loneliness and fortifying emotional resilience.

High-quality social connections serve as effective stress buffers, exerting a positive impact on physical health outcomes. A varied social network plays a role in enhancing physical well-being by fostering a supportive environment that facilitates effective stress management.

Establishing meaningful, high-quality connections has been correlated with extended longevity and enhanced overall health outcomes. Research indicates that the quantity of social connections is associated with decreased mortality rates and improved health across diverse populations.

In times of crisis, the quality of social connections becomes crucial, offering effective coping mechanisms and emotional sustenance. A greater quantity of social connections enhances resilience by providing a range of perspectives and diverse support systems.

Profound connections play a pivotal role in personal growth, nurturing a sense of security that empowers individuals to explore their potential. A varied social network promotes ongoing learning and personal development by introducing individuals to innovative ideas and experiences.

Cultural norms can influence the emphasis placed on either the quality or quantity of social connections, shaping individual expectations for well-being. Recognising the diversity of individual preferences, some may find fulfilment in a few high-quality connections, while others thrive in a larger, more diverse network.

Online connections can enhance well-being when they involve authentic and meaningful interactions. Social media and technology empower individuals to maintain a greater quantity of connections, although the depth of these connections may vary. Analysing the influence of both the quality and quantity of social connections on well-being highlights the intricate and interrelated nature of social dynamics.

Recognising and tackling the adverse effects of loneliness and social isolation on mental health is essential for fostering overall well-being. Loneliness is the subjective experience of feeling alone or disconnected, even in the company of others. On the other hand, social isolation denotes the objective condition of having limited social contact or engagement with others. Persistent loneliness heightens the risk of developing depression and anxiety disorders.

Loneliness is correlated with heightened stress levels and increased cortisol production, exerting a negative impact on mental health. Long-term loneliness has been associated with cognitive decline and an elevated risk of conditions such as Alzheimer's disease. Social isolation can lead to structural changes in the brain, particularly in areas related to memory and cognition. Additionally, loneliness may contribute to lower self-esteem and a diminished sense of self-worth.

Individuals grappling with loneliness may develop pessimistic views about themselves and their capacity to forge meaningful connections. Loneliness has been linked to a heightened risk of cardiovascular diseases, emphasising the intricate link between mental and physical health. Social isolation can compromise the immune system, rendering individuals more vulnerable to illnesses. Chronic loneliness is connected to an increased risk of suicidal ideation and self-harm. Feelings of isolation can escalate mental health crises, precipitating severe consequences.

Taking an active role in community activities and events nurtures social connections. Involvement in volunteer work not only offers opportunities for social interaction but also contributes to a sense of purpose. Joining clubs or groups aligned with personal interests facilitates the development of shared connections.

Embracing technology for virtual socialisation helps bridge physical gaps and sustains connections. Participation in online communities enables individuals to connect with like-minded people, overcoming geographical constraints. Seeking therapy or counselling offers a supportive and confidential space to address feelings of loneliness.

Participating in support groups, whether in-person or online, links individuals with others facing similar challenges. Prioritising a few profound and meaningful connections over numerous superficial relationships elevates the quality of social interactions. Engaging in honest and open communication with friends, family, or colleagues nurtures a supportive network.

Tackling the adverse effects of loneliness and social isolation on mental health necessitates a comprehensive approach. Recognising the interconnectedness of mental and physical health, implementing strategies to cultivate meaningful connections, and seeking professional support when necessary are crucial steps. By actively addressing and mitigating loneliness, individuals can significantly contribute to their mental well-being and overall quality of life.

Immerse yourself completely in social interactions to nurture authentic connections. Hone persuasive communication skills, encompassing active listening, empathy, and assertiveness. Acquire the ability to initiate and sustain conversations, effectively breaking the ice in social settings. Create regular routines for social activities, ensuring consistent opportunities for connection. Strike a balance between social engagement and personal downtime to ward off burnout. Cultivate an inclusive attitude, trying to involve others in social activities.

Contribute to the establishment of inclusive spaces that foster a sense of welcome and acceptance for individuals. Enrolling in educational programs or classes facilitates the creation of connections through shared learning experiences. Acquiring new skills in a group setting not only encourages social interaction but also promotes collaboration. Combating loneliness and enhancing social connectedness requires a combination of self-awareness, proactive engagement, and the cultivation of strong social skills.

Appreciating the impact of cultural and diversity factors on relationships is essential for promoting inclusivity, respect, and effective communication. It's crucial to explore the multifaceted dimensions of how culture and diversity contribute to shaping relationships.

Various cultures highlight unique values, such as collectivism, individualism, hierarchy, or egalitarianism, which in turn influence the dynamics of relationships. Individual identities are frequently intricately connected to cultural backgrounds, shaping perspectives on both self and others.

Nurturing cultural sensitivity is essential for comprehending and respecting differences within relationships. Open and honest communication regarding cultural expectations and differences serves to build mutual understanding. Cultural backgrounds play a significant role in shaping approaches to conflict resolution, with some cultures leaning towards direct confrontation while others value indirect resolution.

Developing cultural competence equips individuals to navigate conflicts stemming from cultural differences. Parents hailing from diverse cultural backgrounds for instance, may encounter challenges in raising children with a multicultural identity.

Cultural competence and inclusivity stand as essential elements in cultivating robust connections, fostering understanding, and nurturing respectful relationships across diverse backgrounds. Cultural competence entails being aware, sensitive, and respectful of cultural differences, thereby nurturing the ability to interact effectively with individuals from diverse backgrounds.

Nurturing cultural competence is a continuous endeavour that demands a dedication to acquiring knowledge about various cultures, customs, and perspectives. Acknowledging and questioning stereotypes associated with distinct cultures is a pivotal step in the development of cultural competence.

Stereotypes can impede understanding, cultural competence dismantles these barriers, fostering more authentic and open connections. Inclusivity encompasses the embrace and appreciation of diversity in all its forms, be it related to culture, race, ethnicity, gender, or other dimensions.

Inclusivity establishes environments where individuals can express their identities safely, free from the apprehension of judgment or discrimination. Cultural competence enhances communication by promoting active listening and sensitivity to verbal and nonverbal cues from diverse perspectives.

Ensuring that communication is effective across cultures, inclusivity works to minimise misunderstandings and misinterpretations. Cultural competence, in turn, cultivates an appreciation for diverse viewpoints, fostering respect for the distinctive qualities that each person contributes to a connection.

Inclusivity requires avoiding assumptions grounded in stereotypes and approaching individuals with an open mind. Cultural competence amplifies adaptability, enabling individuals to navigate diverse cultural contexts seamlessly. Inclusivity plays a role in cultivating robust people skills, forging connections that transcend cultural barriers. Cultural competence establishes trust by highlighting dependability and reliability in cross-cultural interactions.

Inclusivity nurtures authenticity, urging individuals to engage in genuine and transparent interactions. Cultural competence elevates conflict resolution skills, empowering individuals to navigate disagreements and misunderstandings with sensitivity.

Encouraging open dialogue about cultural differences, inclusivity establishes an environment where individuals feel at ease discussing and understanding diverse perspectives. Cultural competence holds significant importance in professional settings, contributing to the success of diverse teams and fostering a harmonious work environment.

Professionals possessing cultural competence are in high demand due to their ability to effectively engage with a diverse spectrum of clients, colleagues, and stakeholders. Integrating cultural competence into educational curricula is crucial for preparing individuals for a globalised world. In educational institutions, inclusivity initiatives cultivate cultural awareness and instil a sense of social responsibility.

Cultural competence extends to community engagement, where celebrations of diversity and inclusivity contribute to strengthening the social fabric. Collaborative endeavours between different communities further the cause of inclusivity and cross-cultural understanding.

Cultural competence and inclusivity transcend mere buzzwords, they are foundational principles that support robust and flourishing connections. Embracing these principles enables individuals and communities to cultivate environments where everyone feels acknowledged, listened to, and respected. This, in turn, contributes to a world teeming with diverse and meaningful relationships.

The swift evolution of technology has profoundly altered how individuals establish, sustain, and encounter relationships in today's society. The rise of smartphones, social media, and messaging apps has revolutionised communication, offering instant connectivity regardless of geographical distances.

Despite facilitating swift and continuous communication, technology introduces challenges, such as the misinterpretation of messages and potential distractions. In long-distance relationships, technology empowers individuals to uphold a sense of closeness through video calls, messaging, and shared digital experiences.

However, challenges like time zone differences and dependence on digital communication tools can influence the depth of connection. Social media platforms provide a means for individuals to share their lives, connect with friends, and expand social circles by meeting new people.

Conversely, the overuse of social media can contribute to social comparison, affecting both self-esteem and relationships. Technology has simplified the process of meeting potential partners through online dating platforms, expanding the dating pool. However, the selective portrayal of identities online can pose challenges in establishing authentic connections.

Technology enables couples to express intimacy through text messages, video calls, and the sharing of digital content. While augmenting connection, maintaining a balance between digital and in-person intimacy is essential for the health of the relationship.

In the digital age, preserving privacy becomes challenging as relationships become increasingly visible through shared photos, posts, and online interactions. Excessive sharing and constant connectivity may result in trust issues, underscoring the need for open communication about boundaries.

Parenting in the digital era requires addressing challenges related to screen time, online safety, and sustaining family connections. The surge in remote work, facilitated by technology, presents challenges in maintaining a clear boundary between work and personal life.

Striking a balance in technology use is essential for preserving quality time with family and ensuring a healthy work-life balance. While the integration of smart devices into homes offers convenience, it also prompts questions about privacy and potential impacts on family dynamics.

Dependence on smart devices might lead to a decline in face-to-face interactions, affecting the depth of relationships. Excessive technology use, often termed tech addiction, can result in diminished face-to-face interactions, thereby impacting the quality of relationships.

Cultivating healthy screen time habits is paramount for sustaining meaningful connections in the digital age. The digital landscape introduces fresh challenges, including cyber threats, underscoring the significance of cybersecurity in safeguarding personal information and relationships.

Establishing and upholding trust in online interactions is essential for the overall well-being of relationships. Ethical considerations in the digital realm involve respecting online boundaries, consent, and preserving integrity in online interactions. Navigating the digital world with responsibility and ethical awareness contributes to the development of healthier relationships, both online and offline.

As technology advances, its integration into relationships will evolve, offering both opportunities and challenges. Couples and individuals must adapt, engage in open communication about technology use, and set boundaries to nurture healthy relationships in the digital era. The impact of technology on relationships is multifaceted, introducing both advantages and complexities.

While technology facilitates connection and communication, deliberate management is necessary to uphold the depth, trust, and intimacy that define healthy relationships. Striking a balance between the benefits and challenges of technology is crucial for navigating the ever-changing landscape of relationships in the digital age.

Robust relationships are constructed upon the bedrock of individual well-being. Accentuating the importance of self-care is vital for upholding emotional, mental, and physical health within the realm of relationships. Prioritising self-care guarantees that individuals approach relationships from a position of strength and self-fulfilment. Consistent self-care practices foster resilience, empowering individuals to navigate challenges within relationships with increased ease.

Sufficient sleep, consistent exercise, and a well-balanced diet form integral element of physical self-care. Involvement in activities that enhance mental and emotional well-being, such as mindfulness, therapy, and hobbies, cultivates emotional resilience.

Nurturing connections with friends and participating in social activities contribute to a robust social support system. Exploring one's beliefs, values, and spiritual practices instils a sense of purpose and fulfilment. Prioritising self-care equips individuals to bring a sense of fulfilment to a relationship, fostering both individual and collective growth.

Self-care acts as a safeguard against the pitfalls of co-dependency by promoting autonomy and individual growth within a relationship. Consistent self-care amplifies communication skills, as individuals become more attuned to their needs and can articulate them effectively. Setting and maintaining boundaries, a fundamental aspect of self-care, contributes to a balanced and respectful relationship dynamic.

Self-care equips individuals with coping mechanisms to navigate stressors, averting the adverse effects of personal challenges on a relationship. During shared moments of stress, those who prioritise self-care can offer each other more effective support. Self-care encourages self-reflection, fostering emotional intelligence and a deeper understanding of one's own and others' emotions. Emotional intelligence gained through self-care enhances empathy and compassion, crucial elements for healthy relationship dynamics.

Instituting daily self-care rituals, whether through morning routines, exercise, or mindfulness practices, establishes a positive tone for the day. Regular self-assessment and check-ins ensure a continuous awareness of personal needs, allowing for adjustments to self-care practices. Seeking therapy or counselling as a form of self-care equips individuals with valuable tools for navigating personal challenges and fostering growth within a relationship.

Emphasising the significance of self-care in sustaining healthy relationships becomes an investment in the well-being of individuals and the reciprocity that contributes to the growth and longevity of the relationship.

Striking a balance between individual well-being and the health of the relationship is crucial for cultivating harmony and longevity. Individual well-being commences with self-discovery, encompassing an understanding of one's needs, values, and personal growth aspirations. Encouraging individuals to pursue their personal passions and interests adds to their sense of fulfilment and happiness.

A thriving relationship is marked by mutual growth, with all parties supporting each other's aspirations and contributing to shared goals. Establishing open lines of communication nurtures, a supportive environment for discussing individual needs within the relationship.

Achieving a balance between interdependence and independence is crucial, enabling shared experiences while respecting individual space and autonomy. Interdependence entails relying on each other for emotional support and collaboration, bolstering the strength of the relationship.

Open communication about individual needs ensures that all parties feel heard and understood. Demonstrating empathy and compassion towards each other's pursuits creates an environment where individual achievements are celebrated.

Establishing collective goals fosters a sense of unity and purpose within a relationship. Identifying shared values aids in establishing common ground for mutual aspirations. Respecting individual differences is crucial for a healthy relationship, allowing for the appreciation of each other's unique qualities. Supporting individual growth, even if it results in changes within the relationship dynamic, is an investment in long-term happiness.

Marking individual and shared successes serves to strengthen the relationship bond and cultivate a positive environment. Approaching conflicts with a constructive mindset permits for the resolution of individual concerns while upholding the health of the relationship. Delving into the root of individual concerns during conflicts contributes to the discovery of mutually beneficial solutions. Embracing flexibility and adaptability ensures a smoother navigation through life changes, accommodating individual growth trajectories.

In the ever-evolving landscape of individuals and relationships, adapting to new dynamics ensures ongoing harmony and satisfaction. Regularly reassessing the equilibrium between individual well-being and the overall health of the relationship permits necessary adjustments. Mutual respect stands as the foundational element underlying the balance between individual and collective needs. It ensures that decisions and actions consider both individual and collective well-being, fostering a harmonious relationship.

Maintaining a robust and enduring relationship necessitates commitment, effort, and a proactive approach to tackle challenges. The establishment of open and honest communication is pivotal for comprehending each other's needs, resolving conflicts, and preserving emotional intimacy.

Chapter 10 - The Impact of Environmental Factors on Longevity

The relationship between the environment and human health is a dynamic and intricate relationship that significantly influences the duration and quality of life. As we navigate the complexities of modern existence, an increasing body of research underscores the profound impact environmental factors have on longevity. From the air we breathe to the water we consume, the places we inhabit, and the broader climate we experience, the environment shapes our health in profound ways.

This chapter delves into the multifaceted dimensions of the impact of environmental factors on longevity, seeking to unravel the intricate connection between our surroundings and the duration of our existence. Understanding these relationships is not only pivotal for individual well-being but also crucial in formulating strategies for sustainable living that foster both human health and the health of our planet.

The influence of air pollution on life expectancy is a critical aspect of environmental health, reflecting the sophisticated relationship between the quality of the air we breathe and our overall well-being. Air pollution, primarily driven by human activities such as industrial processes, transportation, and energy production, introduces a myriad of pollutants into the atmosphere. Among these pollutants, fine particulate matter (PM2.5), nitrogen dioxide (NO2), sulphur dioxide (SO2), and ozone (O3) are prominent contributors to adverse health effects.

Inhaling air pollutants poses a significant threat to respiratory well-being, intensifying ailments like asthma and chronic obstructive pulmonary disease (COPD). Prolonged exposure to air pollution is associated with an elevated likelihood of developing cardiovascular diseases, such as heart attacks and strokes.

Some air pollutants fall into the category of carcinogens, playing a role in the emergence of lung cancer and other respiratory malignancies. Vulnerable demographic groups, particularly children facing developmental challenges and the elderly encountering heightened cardiovascular risks, are particularly susceptible to the health ramifications of air pollution.

Dwelling predominantly in regions marked by heightened pollution, economically disadvantaged communities confront an uneven burden on their health, exacerbated by restricted access to healthcare resources. The swift pace of urbanisation amplifies air pollution levels, particularly in densely populated locales characterised by heavy vehicular traffic and industrial pursuits.

Certain pollutants, such as black carbon, play a role in climate change, hastening the thawing of ice and snow. The enforcement of rigorous air quality standards and regulatory interventions stands as a pivotal strategy to curtail emissions originating from both industries and vehicles.

Shifting towards cleaner energy alternatives and endorsing sustainable transportation stands as an effective strategy to alleviate the origins of air pollution. Elevating public consciousness regarding the health repercussions of air pollution serves to motivate individuals towards embracing cleaner habits and championing environmental policies.

Enlisting community participation in monitoring air quality and championing green initiatives empowers local endeavours aimed at pollution reduction. Progress in air purification technologies presents remedies for indoor environments, augmenting air quality and diminishing personal exposure. The integration of technologies curbing emissions from industrial operations and vehicles contributes significantly to reducing overall ambient pollution levels.

The significance of pristine air in fostering a longer lifespan constitutes a crucial facet of environmental health, underscoring the far-reaching influence that air quality wields over general well-being and life expectancy. Defined by minimal levels of pollutants and contaminants, clean air becomes indispensable for upholding respiratory health and warding off an array of diseases. Its pivotal role extends to the prevention of respiratory ailments like asthma, bronchitis, and chronic obstructive pulmonary disease (COPD).

Diminishing airborne pollutants serves to decrease the likelihood of respiratory infections and complications, especially among susceptible demographics like children and the elderly. Elevated air quality correlates with a diminished risk of cardiovascular diseases, encompassing heart attacks and strokes. Pristine air actively contributes to enhanced blood vessel function, decreased inflammation, and, in turn, bolsters overall cardiovascular health.

Extended exposure to pristine air is associated with a diminished risk of respiratory cancers, notably lung cancer. Diminished levels of air pollutants foster a healthier environment, creating conditions less favourable for the formation of cancerous cells. Beyond its impact on physical health, clean air exerts positive effects on cognitive function and mental well-being, thereby reducing the susceptibility to neurodegenerative diseases.

Elevated air quality is linked to reduced rates of cognitive decline and a decreased occurrence of conditions such as Alzheimer's disease. Moreover, clean air actively supports a robust immune system, bolstering the body's capacity to ward off infections and diseases.

Minimising exposure to pollutants enhances immune function, thereby promoting overall health and longevity. Expectant mothers breathing clean air create a more favourable environment for the development of the foetus, consequently lowering the risk of complications.

Children brought up in regions with pristine air exhibit improved lung development and a reduced susceptibility to respiratory problems. Extended exposure to clean air correlates with an elevated quality of life, nurturing both physical well-being and psychological health. Individuals residing in areas characterised by good air quality are prone to encountering fewer health-related constraints, paving the way for a more active and fulfilling life.

The advocacy for clean air policies plays a pivotal role in establishing fair living conditions for everyone, regardless of socio-economic backgrounds. Endeavours to uphold clean air standards are intertwined with the larger mission of tackling climate change, as the reduction of emissions proves beneficial to both environmental well-being and human health. Initiatives aimed at ensuring clean air align seamlessly with broader sustainability objectives, fostering a healthier planet for both present and future generations.

In the pursuit of extending life expectancy, acknowledging the crucial influence of clean air on health emerges as imperative. Holistic approaches that involve air quality regulations, sustainable urban planning, and public awareness campaigns play a vital role in shaping environments that not only contribute to longer lives but also foster healthier and more vibrant ones.

The impact of water pollution on both health and longevity is substantial, given the material risks posed by contaminated water sources to individuals and communities. This pollution stems from diverse sources, encompassing industrial discharges, agricultural runoff, improper waste disposal, and insufficient sanitation. Within contaminated water, pathogens like bacteria, viruses, and parasites thrive, giving rise to waterborne diseases. Among the prevalent illnesses are diarrhoea, cholera, dysentery, giardiasis, and typhoid fever, presenting as severe and potentially life-threatening, particularly among vulnerable populations.

Ensuring access to clean water is essential for the well-being of both mothers and children. Waterborne diseases pose significant threats during pregnancy, heightening the chances of infant mortality. Contaminated water sources play a role in transmitting infections to infants, jeopardising their health and longevity.

Extended exposure to water pollutants, including heavy metals like lead and mercury, as well as industrial chemicals, is linked to the development of chronic health conditions. Prolonged exposure may result in conditions such as kidney damage, liver disease, developmental issues in children, and an elevated risk of cancer.

The intake of water tainted by pollutants has the potential to undermine the immune system, heightening vulnerability to infections and illnesses. A compromised immune system diminishes the body's capacity to combat diseases, exerting a profound impact on overall health and potentially curtailing lifespan. Water pollution, in addition to its direct effects, can result in the release of airborne pollutants during water treatment procedures, thus playing a role in the development of respiratory issues.

Prolonged exposure to these contaminants may yield uncertain health effects, influencing individuals over an extended duration. The repercussions of water pollution extend to aquatic ecosystems, resulting in the contamination of fish and other seafood. The consumption of contaminated seafood introduces pollutants into the human body, giving rise to health concerns and potentially diminishing lifespan. Notably, water pollution disproportionately impacts vulnerable populations, exacerbating existing social and economic inequalities.

The absence of clean water access perpetuates a cycle of poverty, curtailing opportunities for education, employment, and overall well-being. Water pollution further fuels water scarcity, heightening competition for clean water resources. Resulting water-related conflicts can trigger displacement, disrupt livelihoods, and adversely affect the health and lifespan of affected communities.

This issue of water pollution transcends borders, posing a global health challenge that both developed and developing countries grapple with. International collaboration emerges as imperative to address transboundary water pollution and its far-reaching impact on global health and longevity.

The importance of having access to clean water for a longer and healthier life cannot be overstated. The availability of safe and uncontaminated water is fundamental to preserving human health and well-being. Clean water is vital for numerous physiological functions, preventing diseases, and enhancing overall quality of life.

The importance of clean water extends beyond mere hydration, it is essential for supporting critical physiological functions like digestion, nutrient absorption, and temperature regulation. Adequate hydration is a cornerstone of overall well-being, safeguarding against health issues associated with dehydration that could potentially undermine longevity. The availability of clean water stands as a pivotal factor in warding off waterborne diseases triggered by pathogenic microorganisms prevalent in contaminated water sources.

The presence of contaminated water can result in gastrointestinal problems, malnutrition, and a general compromise of health, thereby affecting longevity. Access to clean water serves to mitigate the risk of chronic health conditions linked to exposure to waterborne pollutants like heavy metals and industrial chemicals.

Populations with access to clean water exhibit lower prevalence rates of chronic conditions such as kidney disease, liver damage, and cancers. Proper hydration with clean water fosters a resilient immune system, enhancing the body's ability to defend against infections and diseases. The availability of clean water plays a role in bolstering overall health resilience, potentially extending life expectancy.

The consumption of clean water for hydration correlates with enhanced cognitive function and mental well-being. Having access to clean water diminishes the likelihood of mental health issues associated with dehydration, thereby contributing to a life that is both healthier and more fulfilling.

The availability of clean water carries economic and social implications, empowering individuals to lead more productive lives. Redirecting the time spent fetching water, particularly by women and children in various communities, towards pursuits like education, work, and other activities fosters social and economic development.

The importance of clean water in agriculture cannot be overstated, as it plays a vital role in cultivating safe and nutritious food. Employing sustainable water practices in agriculture not only ensures food security but also encourages a balanced diet, exerting a positive influence on the health and longevity of communities.

The availability of clean water doesn't just contribute to agricultural needs, it also strengthens community resilience against the effects of climate change, including droughts and extreme weather events. Consistent access to clean water serves as a crucial support system for communities in adapting to environmental challenges, thereby safeguarding both health and well-being.

Climate conditions exert a substantial influence on life expectancy, shaping health outcomes, disease patterns, and overall well-being. The complex relationship between climate and human health encompasses multiple factors, including temperature variations, air quality, occurrences of extreme weather events, and the prevalence of infectious diseases.

Extended exposure to extreme heat can result in heat-related illnesses, cardiovascular issues, and dehydration, with elevated risks for vulnerable populations, particularly the elderly and those with pre-existing health conditions.

Extreme cold temperatures heighten the susceptibility to respiratory diseases, cardiovascular events, and hypothermia, especially in regions lacking sufficient heating infrastructure. Elevated concentrations of air pollutants, encompassing particulate matter and ground-level ozone, are associated with respiratory diseases, cardiovascular issues, and premature mortality. Shifts in climate conditions can alter the frequency and distribution of respiratory infections, influencing mortality rates, particularly in areas with vulnerable populations.

Shifts in climate conditions influence the distribution and behaviour of disease vectors like mosquitoes and ticks, contributing to the transmission of diseases such as malaria, dengue fever, and Lyme disease. Alterations in temperature and precipitation patterns have the potential to broaden the geographical reach of vector-borne diseases, exposing populations that were previously unaffected and affecting life expectancy.

Areas grappling with water scarcity because of climate change may encounter difficulties in upholding proper hygiene and sanitation practices, thereby contributing to the proliferation of waterborne diseases.

The inundation caused by floods and hurricanes has the potential to pollute water sources, resulting in the emergence of waterborne diseases such as cholera and dysentery, impacting both immediate and prolonged health. Variability in climate patterns directly affects crop yields, influencing the availability and nutritional quality of food.

Alterations in temperature and precipitation patterns may precipitate food shortages, compromising the nutritional content of staple crops and contributing to malnutrition, thereby influencing life expectancy. Exposure to extreme weather events, including hurricanes, floods, and wildfires, can be a catalyst for mental health issues such as anxiety, depression, and post-traumatic stress disorder (PTSD).

The displacement and migration triggered by climate changes can result in social and economic upheavals, adding to the mental health challenges faced by affected communities. Climate conditions have the potential to worsen existing chronic health issues, particularly respiratory and cardiovascular diseases.

The heightened occurrence and intensity of heatwaves contribute to elevated mortality rates, especially in regions lacking sufficient infrastructure to cope with extreme heat. Vulnerable populations, such as low-income communities and marginalised groups, often bear a disproportionate burden of the impacts of climate conditions. Disruptions stemming from climate-related events can impede access to healthcare, amplifying prevailing health disparities and differentially affecting life expectancy across diverse populations.

In regions marked by prolonged life expectancies, a harmonious interplay of numerous factors contributes to the enduring health and well-being of their residents. Several pivotal elements work in concert, fostering a comprehensive and supportive environment that sustains longevity. The rationale behind the extended life expectancies in these areas encompasses a spectrum of interconnected factors.

The foundation of regions boasting extended life expectancies lies in their robust and accessible healthcare systems. Well-established medical facilities, comprehensive preventive care programs, and efficient healthcare delivery collectively enhance the overall health of the population.

Proactive public health initiatives, which encompass vaccination programs, disease prevention campaigns, and health education, play a pivotal role in this equation. These initiatives significantly contribute to both the prevention and early detection of illnesses, thereby positively influencing life expectancy.

Regions characterised by extended life expectancies frequently highlight healthful dietary habits. Diets abundant in fruits, vegetables, whole grains, and lean proteins not only support overall health but also diminish the risk of chronic diseases, fostering longevity. Embracing healthy lifestyle choices, including regular physical activity, minimal tobacco and alcohol consumption, and effective stress management, plays a substantial role.

These regions often prioritise a well-balanced approach to life, cultivating habits that enhance well-being. Robust social support networks and active community engagement are prevalent in regions with extended life expectancies. These social connections contribute to mental well-being, alleviate stress, and provide a safety net that positively influences longevity.

Elevated levels of education and widespread health awareness are pivotal factors in fostering informed decision-making about personal health. Educated populations tend to embrace healthier lifestyles and proactively seek timely medical care, thereby positively influencing life expectancy. Economic stability also plays a crucial role in ensuring access to healthcare, education, and maintaining a high standard of living.

Regions characterised by longer life expectancies often showcase economic prosperity, consequently reducing disparities in health outcomes. Additionally, a clean and sustainable environment is conducive to health. Regions prioritising environmental conservation and maintaining low pollution levels contribute significantly to respiratory health and overall well-being.

Cultural practices emphasising a holistic and balanced approach to life wield a notable influence on longevity. The incorporation of mindfulness, traditional healing methods, and a robust sense of community in these practices contributes significantly to overall health. Although genetics play a role, their influence is intricately woven with lifestyle and environmental factors.

Regions boasting extended life expectancies may indeed display favourable genetic predispositions, yet the pivotal role of lifestyle choices cannot be overstated. Forward-thinking government policies, encompassing social welfare programs, healthcare subsidies, and regulations fostering a healthy environment, play a crucial part in enhancing the overall well-being of the population.

The influence of healthcare accessibility on longevity stands as a vital facet of public health and overall well-being. Directly affecting the prevention, early detection, and management of health conditions. Access to healthcare services plays a pivotal role in determining the length of life.

When healthcare is accessible, individuals can undergo regular check-ups and screenings, facilitating the early detection of potential health issues. Additionally, timely access to vaccination programs aids in preventing the spread of infectious diseases, thereby reducing the likelihood of severe illnesses, and enhancing overall health.

Accessible healthcare is a linchpin for individuals with chronic conditions, facilitating continuous monitoring and management to prevent complications and enhance life expectancy. Consistent access to medications and treatment plans holds paramount importance for those with chronic diseases, ensuring proper adherence and disease control.

The immediate availability of emergency care services is vital for addressing acute health issues, accidents, and injuries, thereby averting fatalities. Swift diagnosis and timely interventions in cases of serious illnesses contribute significantly to improved treatment outcomes and heightened life expectancy.

Ensuring access to maternal healthcare services is pivotal for the well-being of both mothers and infants, diminishing the risk of complications during pregnancy and childbirth. Healthcare accessibility plays a crucial role in supporting child immunisation programs, curbing the spread of infectious diseases, and fostering the health of young populations.

Accessible mental health services make substantial contributions to overall well-being, mitigating the impact of mental health issues on physical health and enhancing life expectancy. Timely intervention and support for mental health challenges play a vital role in preventing suicidal behaviours, thereby exerting a positive influence on longevity.

Healthcare accessibility encompasses educational initiatives aimed at promoting health awareness and preventive measures, empowering individuals to make informed decisions about their well-being. Public health campaigns with a focus on disease prevention and lifestyle modifications contribute to fostering a healthier population and ultimately increasing life expectancy. The assurance of equitable access to healthcare services plays a crucial role in reducing disparities in health outcomes among various socio-economic and demographic groups.

Technological innovations, notably telemedicine, broaden the accessibility of healthcare, particularly in remote or underserved areas, leading to improvements in overall health outcomes. Accessible electronic health records facilitate seamless communication between healthcare providers, ensuring coordinated and effective care. Substantial investment in healthcare infrastructure, encompassing hospitals, clinics, and medical facilities, not only enhances accessibility but also contributes to overall improvements in health outcomes.

Discrimination and bias within the healthcare system may lead to disparate treatment, impacting the quality of care received by specific individuals or groups. Encountering discrimination in healthcare settings can result in stress, anxiety, and hesitancy to seek medical care, detrimentally affecting health outcomes.

Disparities in diabetes care, influenced by race and socio-economic factors, contribute to variations in outcomes, encompassing complications and mortality. Inequities in cardiovascular care and preventive measures further give rise to discrepancies in heart disease outcomes and life expectancy. The COVID-19 pandemic has underscored healthcare disparities, with certain communities experiencing elevated infection rates, severe outcomes, and increased mortality.

Addressing healthcare disparities entails the implementation of policies that champion equitable access to care, augment health literacy, nurture cultural competence within the healthcare workforce, and address social determinants of health. Through the alleviation of these disparities, societies can strive towards attaining health equity, ultimately enhancing overall life expectancy for all individuals.

The impact of food security and malnutrition on longevity is substantial, exerting influence on the health and well-being of individuals and populations. Access to ample, nutritious food stands as a fundamental determinant of life expectancy. Ensuring adequate food security guarantees consistent access to a varied array of nutrient-rich foods, thereby fostering overall health and longevity.

The pivotal role of food security lies in averting undernutrition, which, if unaddressed, can give rise to various health issues and affect life expectancy. Inadequate intake of calories, proteins, and essential nutrients can lead to undernutrition, resulting in stunted growth, weakened immune system, and heightened susceptibility to diseases.

Consuming excessive amounts of unhealthy foods, commonly linked to high-calorie and low-nutrient diets, plays a role in the development of obesity and associated health issues, impacting longevity. Insufficient intake of crucial micronutrients, such as vitamins and minerals, can give rise to diverse health problems, including anaemia, vision impairment, and compromised immune function. Malnutrition further weakens the immune system, heightening susceptibility to infections and diminishing the ability to recover from illnesses.

Insufficient nutrition during pregnancy may lead to low birth weight, preterm births, and developmental challenges, shaping the lifelong health trajectory of the child. Early childhood malnutrition can leave enduring imprints on cognitive development, physical growth, and overall well-being, thereby influencing longevity.

In the broader context, poor nutrition emerges as a contributing factor to the onset of chronic diseases like heart disease, diabetes, and hypertension, all of which can curtail life expectancy. Conversely, overnutrition and unhealthy dietary patterns contribute to obesity, elevating the risk of obesity-related conditions and diminishing life expectancy.

Malnutrition is frequently encountered among the elderly, influencing their overall health, immune function, and vulnerability to infections, consequently impacting life expectancy. Insufficient access to nutritious food in low-income countries contributes to malnutrition in children, affecting growth and influencing long-term health outcomes.

In numerous developing nations, food insecurity arises from poverty, constraining access to a variety of nutrient-dense foods essential for sustaining health and longevity. The weakened immune system resulting from malnutrition renders individuals more susceptible to infectious diseases prevalent in resource-limited settings.

On a global scale, discrepancies in access to nutritious food play a role in the divergent life expectancies observed across various regions and populations. Socioeconomic factors wield influence over the accessibility of quality food, presenting greater challenges for marginalised populations in maintaining adequate nutrition. Public health campaigns and nutrition education programs have a goal to heighten awareness about the significance of a balanced diet and its consequential impact on longevity.

Government policies, encompassing initiatives like food assistance programs and regulations advocating for healthy food choices, assume a pivotal role in tackling issues of food security and malnutrition. The promotion of sustainable and diverse agricultural practices becomes instrumental in fostering long-term food security, guaranteeing a steady and nutritious food supply for populations.

Environmental elements, such as climate change, possess the potential to impact food production, posing challenges to the maintenance of food security and exerting influence on overall health outcomes.

Efforts to address the impact of food security and malnutrition on longevity demand a comprehensive approach. This involves enhancing access to nutritious food, promoting education on healthy dietary practices, and implementing policies that specifically target socioeconomic disparities. Prioritising nutritional well-being can have a positive influence on overall health and life expectancy within societies.

The impact of green spaces on mental and physical health stands as a well-documented phenomenon, underscoring the positive effects of natural environments on overall well-being. Crucial in this regard are green spaces like parks, gardens, and natural landscapes, playing a pivotal role in fostering both mental and physical health. Exposure to these green spaces has been correlated with lower stress levels. Nature, with its calming ambiance, can alleviate both the physiological and psychological effects of stress.

Spending time in green spaces is associated with enhanced mood and reduced symptoms of depression and anxiety. Nature exposure is correlated with the release of mood-enhancing neurotransmitters, notably serotonin. Additionally, green environments have demonstrated the ability to boost cognitive function, leading to improvements in concentration, attention, and creativity.

These spaces further foster outdoor activities like walking, jogging, and sports, thereby contributing to elevated levels of physical activity. Regular exercise, as facilitated by green spaces, is crucial for sustaining physical health.

Access to green spaces is correlated with decreased blood pressure, a lower risk of cardiovascular diseases, and enhanced cardiovascular health. Interacting with nature has been associated with improved immune function, with exposure to green environments fortifying the immune system.

The concept of nature therapy, or ecotherapy, revolves around utilising natural environments as a therapeutic tool. This approach has proven effective in treating various mental health conditions. Green spaces serve as healing environments, where natural elements contribute to a sense of restoration and well-being for individuals in the process of recovering from illnesses or surgeries.

Green spaces frequently function as gathering places, nurturing social interactions and community engagement, which, in turn, contribute to both mental and physical health. Communities endowed with access to green spaces often exhibit elevated levels of social cohesion, fostering a sense of belonging and support.

The exposure to nature holds particular significance for the cognitive development of children. Green school environments and outdoor learning spaces have demonstrated positive effects on academic performance and attention span. Children who spend time in these green spaces typically show improved behaviour, diminished symptoms of attention-deficit/hyperactivity disorder (ADHD) and enhanced emotional well-being.

Biophilic design principles revolve around the integration of natural elements into urban and built environments, acknowledging the positive impact of nature on human well-being. The inclusion of greenery in workplaces has been linked to heightened productivity, job satisfaction, and the overall well-being of employees. Green spaces within these environments offer opportunities for restoration, enabling individuals to recuperate from mental fatigue and stress. Exposure to nature plays a role in fostering a sense of relaxation and rejuvenation.

Nature environments, as proposed by the Attention Restoration Theory, provide a rejuvenating experience by enabling individuals to redirect their attention, resulting in enhanced cognitive function. Ensuring fair access to green spaces is vital for promoting health equity. Urban planning that prioritises green infrastructure extends benefits to all residents, regardless of socioeconomic status.

Deprivation of access to green spaces, often termed as nature deprivation, can contribute to detrimental health outcomes. Therefore, initiatives aimed at augmenting the availability of green spaces in urban areas are paramount for public health.

Accumulation of heavy metals in essential organs can result in damage and dysfunction, potentially contributing to premature mortality. Specific chemicals present in consumer products, like phthalates and bisphenol A (BPA), have been associated with endocrine disruption, impacting reproductive health, and potentially influencing lifespan.

Certain chemicals employed in the manufacturing of consumer goods possess carcinogenic properties, heightening the risk of cancer and affecting mortality rates. Extended exposure to ionising radiation, whether stemming from medical procedures, nuclear accidents, or occupational contact, is linked to an increased risk of cancer and other health issues that can impact lifespan.

Excessive exposure to ultraviolet (UV) radiation from the sun stands as a recognised risk factor for skin cancer, with potential implications for longevity. Prolonged exposure to elevated levels of noise pollution has been associated with cardiovascular diseases, including hypertension and heart-related conditions, potentially contributing to a shortened lifespan.

The disruptive effects of noise pollution on sleep patterns can lead to chronic sleep disorders, carrying potential long-term health consequences.

Soil contaminated with pollutants has the potential to contaminate crops, disrupting the food chain and exposing individuals to harmful substances, potentially influencing health and lifespan. Using contaminated soil for agricultural purposes can result in the ingestion of toxic substances, giving rise to a spectrum of health issues.

Some professions entail exposure to hazardous substances like asbestos or industrial chemicals, contributing to occupational diseases, respiratory problems, and heightened mortality risks. The implementation of effective safety measures within workplaces is paramount for minimising exposure to harmful substances and safeguarding the well-being of workers.

Encounters with environmental toxins can exert diverse impacts on both health and lifespan. Managing these risks requires the adoption of sustainable practices, the regulation of harmful substances, and the establishment of policies aimed at shielding individuals from environmental hazards. Essential components in addressing the intricate relationship between environmental toxins and longevity include public awareness, education, and proactive measures.

Prioritising overall health and well-being involves minimising exposure to harmful substances. Stay informed about prevalent harmful elements found in everyday life, including air pollutants, toxins in household products, and contaminants in food and water. Choose organic and natural alternatives in food, personal care products, and household items to diminish exposure to pesticides, synthetic chemicals, and additives.

Promote proper ventilation in living spaces to decrease indoor air pollution. Employ strategies such as opening windows, utilising exhaust fans, and considering air purifiers to enhance overall air quality.

Employ water filters to eliminate contaminants from tap water, particularly in regions where water quality might be a concern. Safeguard food by storing it in secure containers to prevent exposure to harmful substances. Opt for food storage options like glass, stainless steel, or containers made from BPA-free plastic.

Exercise caution in cooking practices to reduce exposure to harmful substances, avoid overheating oils, utilise non-toxic cookware, and choose cooking methods that preserve nutritional value. Reduce reliance on plastic products, especially those containing harmful chemicals like BPA. Instead, embrace reusable and eco-friendly alternatives crafted from glass, stainless steel, or other safe materials.

Choose environmentally friendly and non-toxic cleaning products. Seek out labels that confirm products are devoid of harmful chemicals and contemplate creating homemade cleaning solutions using natural ingredients like vinegar and baking soda. Choose personal care products with minimal or no harmful additives.

Scrutinise labels to recognise and steer clear of ingredients such as parabens, phthalates, and synthetic fragrances. If you cultivate a garden, practice conscientious gardening by refraining from the use of harmful pesticides and fertilisers. Explore organic gardening methods and employ companion planting to naturally manage pests.

Reducing or eliminating alcohol and tobacco consumption can diminish exposure to harmful substances associated with a range of health issues, including cancer and respiratory problems. Incorporate regular health check-ups into your routine to monitor overall health, aiding in the early identification of potential issues related to environmental exposures.

Dispose of hazardous materials, such as electronic waste, batteries, and household chemicals, in accordance with local guidelines to prevent environmental contamination. Practice mindful use of electronics to minimise exposure to electromagnetic radiation, consider using devices in airplane mode, limiting screen time, and establishing electronic-free zones in living spaces.

Embrace and embody sustainable living habits to mitigate overall environmental pollution. Engage in practices such as recycling, waste reduction, and selecting eco-friendly products. Advocate for and endorse policies that regulate and curtail the use of harmful substances. Promote sustainable practices within industries and communities.

Actively participate in community initiatives centred around environmental awareness and sustainability. Contribute to local clean-up endeavours and endorse initiatives dedicated to fostering a healthy environment. When relevant, use personal protective equipment (PPE) to limit exposure to harmful substances, particularly in occupational settings.

The elaborate interplay between socio-economic status (SES) and longevity has undergone thorough examination, revealing a multifaceted phenomenon. SES, comprising elements like income, education, occupation, and resource accessibility, substantially shapes an individual's health outcomes and life expectancy.

Those with elevated socio-economic status commonly enjoy increased access to financial resources, fostering a healthier lifestyle. This encompasses access to nutritious food, quality healthcare, and opportunities for recreational activities.

Elevated educational attainment typically correlates with improved health outcomes and an extended life expectancy. Education empowers individuals with knowledge regarding healthy behaviours, disease prevention, and access to healthcare resources. Occupational status, intertwined with socio-economic status, may expose individuals to varied health risks.

Occupations with higher status often entail superior working conditions, job security, and access to healthcare benefits. The socio-economic status significantly influences healthcare accessibility, with individuals of higher SES more likely to afford quality healthcare, regular check-ups, and preventive measures, thereby enhancing health and longevity.

Socio-economic status shapes lifestyle decisions encompassing diet, physical activity, and substance use. Individuals with higher SES often possess resources to adopt healthier behaviours, diminishing the likelihood of chronic diseases and fostering longevity.

Conversely, lower socio-economic status is frequently linked to heightened stress levels, impacting mental health, and contributing to various health challenges. Chronic stress is associated with conditions like cardiovascular disease, thereby influencing life expectancy.

Elevated socio-economic status correlates with the capacity to establish and sustain robust social support networks. These connections play a pivotal role in enhancing mental well-being and acting as a protective barrier against stress, ultimately contributing to extended longevity. Socio-economic status also exerts an impact on living environments and environmental exposures.

Those with lower SES may inhabit regions with restricted access to green spaces, elevated pollution levels, and insufficient infrastructure, influencing overall health. Additionally, socio-economic status shapes dietary preferences and food security, with higher SES individuals having greater access to diverse and nutritious diets, thereby reducing the risk of malnutrition and related health concerns.

Those with elevated socio-economic status typically enjoy improved access to early interventions, screenings, and preventive healthcare measures. This accessibility to timely healthcare contributes significantly to an extended life expectancy. Socio-economic status frequently exhibits intergenerational continuity, influencing not only an individual's life trajectory but also that of their offspring.

Children born into families with higher SES often benefit from enhanced access to resources, education, and healthcare, establishing a foundation for healthier lives. Discrepancies in socio-economic status contribute to health inequalities, presenting greater obstacles for individuals with lower SES in attaining and sustaining optimal health. Addressing these disparities is imperative for promoting overall longevity.

The trajectory of technological progress holds the capacity to wield both positive and negative repercussions on the environmental elements that shape longevity. Innovations in technology, such as sophisticated sensors and monitoring systems, empower the real-time tracking of environmental variables. This encompasses the monitoring of air and water quality, offering a prospect for early detection of environmental hazards and facilitating prompt interventions to safeguard public health.

The evolution and acceptance of clean energy technologies, exemplified by solar and wind power, have the potential to diminish dependence on fossil fuels. This shift towards cleaner energy sources holds the promise of alleviating air pollution, curbing greenhouse gas emissions, and fostering respiratory well-being, thereby playing a role in augmenting life expectancy.

Agricultural technology, featuring precision farming methodologies and data-centric decision-making, can streamline resource utilisation, curtail environmental repercussions, and bolster the efficiency of food production. The availability of healthier and sustainably cultivated food, in turn, stands as a positive influence on human health and longevity.

Technology plays a pivotal role in advancing environmental conservation endeavours by facilitating streamlined waste management, effective recycling, and sustainable resource utilisation. These conservation initiatives actively contribute to the preservation of biodiversity, the protection of ecosystems, and the cultivation of a healthier environment for communities.

Technology serves as a powerful conduit for environmental education and awareness. Elevated awareness regarding the influence of environmental elements on health can foster enlightened lifestyle decisions, promoting practices conducive to longevity. Computational models and artificial intelligence offer predictive capabilities for environmental risks.

These models enable the anticipation and proactive response to events like natural disasters, disease outbreaks, or pollution incidents, thereby minimising their repercussions on human health. Biotechnological breakthroughs play a crucial role in environmental remediation. Innovations such as bioremediation and genetic engineering have the potential to contribute to the revitalisation of ecosystems impacted by pollution, cultivating healthier living environments.

Innovative water purification technologies, encompassing sophisticated filtration and desalination techniques, offer a pivotal solution for ensuring access to pristine and secure drinking water. This directly attends to a foundational element of human health and longevity. Concurrently, wearable technologies and e-health applications empower individuals to track their personal health metrics. Leveraging this data allows for the early identification of health issues associated with environmental exposures, fostering a proactive approach to health management.

Although technological progress holds considerable promise in addressing environmental challenges, it is imperative to acknowledge potential drawbacks, including the generation of electronic waste, increased energy consumption, and unintended consequences associated with specific technologies. A nuanced and considerate approach to technological innovation becomes paramount to capitalise on the advantages while mitigating adverse effects on both the environment and public health.

Integrate intelligent and eco-friendly transportation systems, encompassing electric vehicles, bike-sharing initiatives, and effective public transit. This not only diminishes air pollution and traffic congestion but also fosters physical activity, fostering healthier communities.

Embrace the tenets of a circular economy to curtail waste production and advocate for sustainable resource utilisation. This entails practices like recycling, upcycling, and minimising single-use items, thereby championing environmental preservation, and cultivating a healthier ecosystem.

Integrate precision farming technologies to streamline resource utilisation in agriculture. Employ data-driven decision-making and satellite imagery to optimise crop yields, minimise pesticide usage, and champion sustainable farming practices.

Harness bioremediation methods for environmental clean-up, engineering microorganisms and plants to absorb and break down pollutants. This contributes to ecosystem restoration, diminishing health risks. Embrace nature-based solutions like reforestation, wetland restoration, and biodiversity conservation to bolster ecosystem services and alleviate the health impacts of climate change.

Enhance healthcare accessibility through the expansion of telehealth services and digital health interventions. Implementing remote monitoring, telemedicine, and health apps can aid in early detection and management of health issues, positively impacting overall longevity. Foster community engagement in environmental initiatives by empowering local communities.

Initiatives like community gardens, clean-up projects, and educational programs contribute to environmental stewardship, fostering community well-being. Develop climate-resilient infrastructure capable of withstanding the impacts of extreme weather events. This involves constructing flood-resistant buildings, implementing improved stormwater management, and adopting sustainable urban planning practices.

Initiate educational campaigns to heighten awareness of the influence of environmental factors on health. Communities equipped with knowledge are more prone to embracing sustainable practices and endorsing policies that uphold environmental and public health. Introduce cutting-edge water management solutions, incorporating water recycling and conservation technologies, to guarantee access to clean water. This approach addresses a pivotal aspect of public health, enhancing longevity.

Advocate for regenerative agriculture practices emphasising soil health, biodiversity, and sustainable farming methods. Nurturing healthy soils not only fosters nutritious food production but also aids in mitigating environmental degradation. Cultivate partnerships between the public and private sectors, academia, and communities to formulate comprehensive solutions. Adopting multidisciplinary approaches allows for the effective addressing of intricate environmental challenges, contributing to overall well-being.

Chapter 11 – The Impact of Finances on Longevity

The relationship between financial stability and longevity is a multifaceted interplay that significantly influences an individual's overall well-being and life expectancy. Beyond the obvious implications of financial resources on accessing healthcare, the impact extends to various dimensions of health, ranging from preventive measures and nutrition to mental well-being and the quality of living environments.

Financial stability enables individuals to make choices that positively contribute to their health, fostering a lifestyle conducive to longevity. This sophisticated connection underscores the importance of addressing economic disparities and promoting financial well-being as integral components of public health initiatives aimed at enhancing longevity and overall quality of life. In this exploration, we delve into the diverse ways in which finances shape health outcomes and contribute to the complex tapestry of factors influencing human longevity.

In the elaborate tapestry of well-being, financial stability emerges as a pivotal thread, weaving its influence across myriad facets of an individual's life. It acts as the cornerstone, allowing individuals the means to embrace regular healthcare services. The tether between financial stability and health insurance is particularly profound, unlocking pathways to essential medical treatments and preventive care, thereby safeguarding one's holistic wellness.

Individuals who enjoy financial stability are inclined to invest in proactive health measures, encompassing vaccinations, screenings, and routine check-ups. Engaging in preventive healthcare not only facilitates the early detection and management of health issues but also lays the foundation for improved long-term outcomes.

Furthermore, financial stability affords enhanced access to nutritious food options, underscoring the pivotal role of economic resources in shaping dietary choices. Recognising the significance of a well-balanced diet, both for maintaining overall health and preventing chronic diseases, accentuates the impact of financial stability on holistic well-being.

Those endowed with financial stability frequently find themselves equipped to partake in physical activities and wellness programs. The availability of gym memberships, fitness classes, and recreational pursuits intertwines with enhanced physical health. Beyond the realm of exercise, financial stability extends its reach, alleviating the stress born from economic uncertainties and insecurities.

Chronic stress, a frequent companion of financial instability, casts a shadow on mental well-being, making financial stability a harbinger of positive mental health outcomes. This equilibrium in financial resources also extends its influence to living conditions, encompassing aspects like housing quality and the choices individuals make regarding their neighbourhoods.

Financial stability serves as a conduit to educational resources, establishing a crucial connection between education and health literacy. This literacy empowers individuals to make discerning choices regarding their health and well-being. Furthermore, financial stability opens the door to participation in social and recreational pursuits, fostering social engagement that, in turn, contributes positively to mental health by diminishing feelings of isolation and loneliness.

Individuals with financial stability often enjoy greater flexibility when it comes to selecting or maintaining employment in environments conducive to well-being. This access to safer working conditions and a reduction in workplace stress exerts a positive influence on their overall health.

Beyond the professional sphere, financial stability permeates various aspects of life, contributing to an elevated quality of life. Those with stable finances are afforded the resources to partake in leisure activities, travel, and other experiences that not only enhance life satisfaction but may also play a role in promoting longevity.

Exploring the intricate connection between economic well-being and longevity reveals a subject of profound significance. Financial stability emerges as a linchpin, intricately shaping multiple dimensions of an individual's health and overall life expectancy. Those with higher economic status tend to enjoy longer and healthier lives.

A salient aspect of this relationship is the capacity to access quality healthcare. Individuals in stable financial positions commonly possess the means to afford routine medical check-ups, preventive screenings, and timely interventions, facilitating early detection and management of health issues.

The sway of economic well-being extends its influence into dietary preferences, with those of higher socioeconomic status typically enjoying improved access to nutritious food choices. A well-rounded diet, fundamental for warding off chronic diseases and upholding overall health, inevitably becomes a determinant of life expectancy.

Beyond dietary considerations, economic status significantly shapes living conditions. Individuals with higher income can secure residences in safer neighbourhoods boasting better air quality, diminished pollution, and enhanced access to green spaces. These elements collectively contribute to fostering a healthier living environment, thereby exerting a positive impact on longevity.

Economic well-being frequently paves the way for access to top-tier education. Elevated education levels correlate with improved health outcomes and an extended life expectancy. Educated individuals typically embrace healthier behaviours and possess a profound understanding of preventive healthcare measures.

Beyond the realm of education, financial stability serves as a buffer against stressors tied to economic insecurity, job instability, and the ability to meet basic needs. This reduction in stress levels becomes a contributing factor to enhanced mental health, thereby exerting a positive influence on overall well-being and longevity.

The nexus between economic well-being and heightened health literacy empowers individuals to make informed decisions about their well-being. This proficiency spans understanding medical information, adhering to treatment plans, and actively participating in preventive health practices.

Interwoven with economic factors are the intricate threads of various social determinants of health, encompassing access to secure housing, quality education, and employment opportunities. This amalgamation of social determinants intricately weaves the complex web of factors that collectively shape and influence life expectancy.

The impact of financial resources on the accessibility of high-quality healthcare stands as a pivotal facet of public health, holding profound implications for individual well-being and overall longevity. In shaping healthcare access, financial resources assume a multifaceted role, exerting influence across various dimensions of the healthcare experience.

The availability of financial resources frequently dictates an individual's capacity to afford health insurance coverage. Those endowed with sufficient financial means can procure comprehensive health insurance plans, encompassing a wider array of medical services, preventive care, and access to a network of healthcare providers. Conversely, uninsured, or underinsured individuals may encounter barriers in accessing essential healthcare services.

The expenses associated with medical services, ranging from doctor's visits and diagnostic tests to medications and surgical procedures, often pose a substantial hurdle for individuals with constrained financial resources. Having adequate financial means empowers individuals to access essential medical treatments without sacrificing necessary care.

Financial stability not only facilitates but encourages active participation in preventive healthcare measures, encompassing routine check-ups, screenings, and vaccinations. Those with financial resources are more inclined to prioritise early detection and prevention, culminating in improved health outcomes and an augmented life expectancy.

Securing access to specialised medical care is frequently contingent on financial resources. Those with elevated incomes often possess the means to consult specialists, undergo advanced diagnostic procedures, and explore innovative treatments. The provision of timely and specialised care can exert a profound influence on individual health trajectories.

Additionally, financial resources wield sway over access to mental health services, encompassing counselling, therapy, and psychiatric care. Recognising mental health as an integral facet of overall well-being, the capacity to afford mental health services plays a pivotal role in fostering improved psychological health and resilience.

The influence of financial stability extends to an individual's choice of residence, impacting access to superior healthcare infrastructure. Those with ample financial resources often opt to reside in areas boasting renowned medical facilities, ensuring convenient access to high-quality healthcare services.

While frequently overlooked, the ability to afford transportation to healthcare facilities is crucial for seamless healthcare access. Financially stable individuals can readily access transportation options, guaranteeing timely arrivals for medical appointments and emergency services.

Another crucial aspect is the affordability of prescription medications, which significantly influences medication adherence. Individuals with financial stability are better equipped to adhere to prescribed medication regimens, effectively averting complications and fostering overall health.

The significance of medical insurance in shaping life expectancy cannot be overstated, as it profoundly influences access to healthcare services, preventive measures, and timely medical interventions. It serves as a facilitator for accessing preventive healthcare services, such as routine check-ups, vaccinations, and screenings. Those covered by insurance are more inclined to participate in proactive health measures, thereby enhancing the likelihood of early detection and prevention of diseases. This focus on preventive care, in turn, fosters better overall health and contributes to increased longevity.

Possessing medical insurance equips individuals with the financial capacity to pursue timely medical interventions when health issues surface. This encompasses swift consultations with healthcare professionals, diagnostic tests, and essential treatments. The significance of prompt medical care lies in its pivotal role in managing and addressing health conditions, averting complications, and ultimately exerting a positive influence on life expectancy.

Moreover, medical insurance frequently encompasses coverage for specialised healthcare services, affording individuals the opportunity to consult specialists, undergo advanced medical procedures, and access tailored treatments. This ensures that individuals can receive the most fitting and effective care tailored to their specific health needs.

Managing chronic conditions, which can wield a significant impact on life expectancy, necessitates continuous attention and treatment. Medical insurance plays a crucial role in facilitating individuals' access to essential medications, therapies, and regular medical appointments, fostering effective management of chronic diseases. The adequacy of this management significantly contributes to improved health outcomes and, consequently, a lengthened life.

Medical insurance serves as a shield against the substantial costs associated with healthcare. Individuals covered by insurance are less prone to encountering financial obstacles when pursuing medical care, diminishing the risk of postponing, or forgoing essential treatments due to economic constraints. This financial safeguard ensures that individuals can access healthcare services without compromising their well-being or life expectancy.

Examining the disparities in health outcomes rooted in socioeconomic status unveils an intricate interplay of diverse factors that wield a profound influence on individuals' well-being and life expectancy. Individuals enjoying elevated socioeconomic status typically benefit from improved access to healthcare resources, encompassing quality medical facilities, specialists, and advanced treatments.

In contrast, those with lower socioeconomic status may encounter barriers to healthcare access, such as limited availability of medical facilities, extended wait times, and challenges in affording medical services.

Those with elevated socioeconomic status frequently embrace healthier lifestyle behaviours, encompassing regular exercise, balanced nutrition, and restrained tobacco and alcohol consumption. Conversely, lower socioeconomic status is correlated with increased rates of unhealthy behaviours, such as smoking, suboptimal diet, and limited physical activity, thereby contributing to a heightened prevalence of chronic diseases.

The affluent population may choose to reside in neighbourhoods characterised by superior environmental conditions, reduced pollution levels, and enhanced access to green spaces, all factors that positively influence overall health. Individuals residing in lower socioeconomic brackets may inhabit areas characterised by elevated environmental pollution, a scarcity of green spaces, and suboptimal living conditions, factors that contribute to health disparities.

Educational attainment emerges as a significant determinant of health outcomes, with higher levels of education being associated with improved well-being. Those with more extensive education typically exhibit heightened health literacy, empowering them to make informed decisions regarding their overall health. Conversely, limited access to education may lead to lower health literacy, posing challenges for individuals in navigating healthcare information, preventive measures, and disease management.

Occupations of higher status typically entail superior working conditions, job security, and access to robust workplace health and safety measures. On the contrary, those in lower-status occupations may contend with occupational hazards, unsafe working conditions, and a restricted access to health and safety resources, consequently heightening health risks.

While higher socioeconomic status may provide financial security, it can also involve high-stress environments. Nevertheless, individuals in higher socioeconomic status groups often enjoy enhanced access to mental health resources.

The economic instability and social stressors linked to lower socioeconomic status contribute to elevated rates of mental health issues, influencing overall well-being. Those with affluence can afford a diverse and nutritious diet, fostering better overall health. Conversely, limited financial resources may give rise to food insecurity, dependence on economical yet less nutritious options, and an increased vulnerability to malnutrition and associated health issues.

Individuals of higher socioeconomic status typically enjoy robust social support networks, a factor that positively influences mental health and contributes to overall well-being. In contrast, limited social support may lead to heightened stress and difficulties in coping with health issues, potentially impacting life expectancy.

Exploring how income inequality may affect life expectancy reveals a nuanced relationship between economic disparities and overall well-being. Individuals in higher income brackets often have better access to quality healthcare, including preventive services, regular check-ups, and advanced medical treatments. Those in lower income groups may face challenges in accessing healthcare due to financial barriers, leading to delayed or insufficient medical care and potential impacts on life expectancy.

Individuals with substantial financial resources typically possess the means to engage in health-promoting behaviours such as regular exercise, maintaining a healthy diet, and participating in wellness programs. This affluence contributes to improved health outcomes.

Conversely, constrained financial resources may lead to unhealthy lifestyle choices, encompassing suboptimal nutrition, insufficient physical activity, and elevated rates of tobacco and alcohol consumption, thereby influencing life expectancy.

Moreover, a higher income often aligns with elevated levels of education. This educational advantage correlates with enhanced health literacy, a greater understanding of disease prevention, and the ability to make informed decisions about one's health. On the contrary, lower income groups may encounter limited access to education, resulting in reduced health literacy. This potential deficit can impact the ability to navigate healthcare systems and adopt health-promoting behaviours.

Professions associated with higher income typically provide improved working conditions, job security, and access to robust workplace safety measures. This reduces the exposure of individuals to occupational health risks. Conversely, those in lower-paying occupations may contend with hazardous working conditions, elevating the risk of occupational diseases and injuries, thereby impacting life expectancy.

Additionally, affluent communities often choose to reside in areas characterised by superior environmental conditions, lower pollution levels, and convenient access to recreational spaces. This positive environment contributes to overall health and well-being. Conversely, lower-income neighbourhoods may encounter heightened levels of environmental pollution, a scarcity of green spaces, and inadequate infrastructure, collectively contributing to health disparities.

Enhanced financial resources frequently correlate with improved living conditions, diminished stress, and expanded access to social support networks, fostering positive effects on mental health and overall well-being. Conversely, economic challenges may elevate stress levels, curtail social support, and introduce adverse social determinants that contribute to health disparities, potentially impacting life expectancy.

Additionally, individuals with affluence can afford a varied and nutritious diet, thereby mitigating the risk of malnutrition and associated health issues. This economic advantage plays a significant role in promoting overall health and well-being.

Constrained financial resources can give rise to food insecurity, dependence on less nutritious options, and an elevated susceptibility to health problems associated with malnutrition. Conversely, affluent individuals often enjoy enhanced access to early interventions, screenings, and preventive healthcare measures, thereby contributing to an augmented life expectancy. Limited resources may lead to delayed or insufficient access to early interventions, potentially influencing health outcomes and longevity.

Exploring the connection between education levels and financial well-being reveals a nuanced interplay of factors that substantially shape an individual's economic status. Those with higher levels of education typically enjoy access to superior job opportunities and avenues for career advancement, ultimately leading to an increased earning potential. Conversely, limited educational qualifications may translate to lower-paying jobs and fewer opportunities for career growth, thereby impacting overall financial well-being.

Earning a higher level of education enhances one's employability and job stability, thereby decreasing the likelihood of experiencing unemployment and periods of financial insecurity. Conversely, limited education may expose individuals to job insecurity, heightened vulnerability during economic downturns, and difficulties in maintaining financial stability.

Education not only imparts academic knowledge but also equips individuals with essential financial literacy skills such as budgeting, investing, and understanding financial markets, contributing to more informed financial decision-making. On the other hand, limited education may result in lower financial literacy, potentially leading to suboptimal money management practices and increased financial stress.

Individuals with advanced education often possess the skills needed to manage debt responsibly, make well-informed financial decisions, and adeptly navigate credit markets. Conversely, limited financial knowledge and education may contribute to elevated levels of debt, encompassing credit card balances and loans, thereby impacting long-term financial well-being.

Education serves as an empowering force, enabling individuals to pursue entrepreneurial ventures and seize opportunities to generate wealth and attain financial success. Conversely, limited education may pose obstacles to entrepreneurial aspirations, restricting access to self-employment opportunities and potential financial prosperity.

Individuals with a solid educational background are more prone to participate in retirement planning, actively contributing to retirement savings and ensuring long-term financial security. Conversely, limited education may lead to inadequate retirement planning, potentially giving rise to financial challenges during the later stages of life.

Educated individuals typically enjoy enhanced access to financial resources, spanning loans, investment opportunities, and financial advice, collectively contributing to their overall financial well-being. On the other hand, limited access to financial resources may translate to a dearth of investment opportunities, reduced financial flexibility, and difficulties in accumulating wealth.

The influence of higher education often manifests positively across subsequent generations, disrupting the cycle of financial instability and fostering a legacy of financial well-being. Conversely, limited education may sustain financial challenges through generations, perpetuating a cycle of economic hardship.

Educated individuals are more inclined to comprehend the significance of health insurance and engage in financial planning for healthcare expenses, thereby contributing to overall financial stability. In contrast, limited education may result in a lack of awareness about financial planning for healthcare, potentially causing financial strain during medical emergencies.

The pursuit of continuous learning and upskilling is prevalent among those with higher education, enabling them to adeptly adapt to changing economic landscapes and uphold financial well-being. On the contrary, limited educational attainment may impede adaptability, posing challenges in navigating evolving job markets and sustaining financial resilience.

The role of education in shaping financial decision-making is a pivotal factor that can profoundly impact an individual's economic well-being and, consequently, their longevity. Education endows individuals with vital financial literacy skills, empowering them to grasp intricate financial concepts or budgets wisely, and make well-informed decisions regarding savings and investments.

Conversely, limited education may give rise to lower financial literacy, leading to difficulties in understanding financial products, effective money management, and making optimal financial decisions.

Individuals with a solid education background are more inclined to participate in comprehensive financial planning, encompassing aspects such as retirement savings and investment strategies. This forward-thinking approach contributes significantly to financial security across various life stages. On the contrary, limited education may steer individuals toward concentrating on short-term financial goals, potentially neglecting long-term planning, and impeding the ability to accumulate wealth for the future.

Education not only equips individuals with financial foresight but also imparts skills for responsible debt management. Educated individuals are more likely to make informed decisions about borrowing, leading to enhanced debt management and reduced financial stress. Conversely, limited financial knowledge may result in suboptimal debt management practices, potentially leading to higher levels of debt and increased financial strain.

Individuals with a solid educational foundation are more apt to comprehend investment opportunities, adeptly manage risks, and grasp the principles of diversification. This understanding facilitates the construction of well-balanced investment portfolios. Conversely, limited education may translate to a lack of comprehension about investment strategies, potentially resulting in suboptimal investment decisions and missed opportunities for accumulating wealth.

Education has the potential to empower individuals to embark on entrepreneurial ventures, opening doors to additional income streams and financial success. Conversely, limited education may curtail entrepreneurial aspirations, constraining the ability to establish alternative sources of income.

Educated individuals typically enjoy improved access to financial resources, spanning loans, credit facilities, and investment opportunities, thereby enhancing financial flexibility. On the contrary, restricted access to financial resources may lead to fewer opportunities for financial growth and an increased dependence on short-term financial solutions.

Education cultivates adaptability to economic changes by imparting skills for lifelong learning and upskilling. This adaptability is essential for navigating dynamic job markets and maintaining financial well-being. Conversely, limited educational attainment may impede adaptability, rendering it challenging to adjust to economic shifts and heightening vulnerability to financial instability.

Educated individuals are more apt to comprehend the significance of health insurance, preventive healthcare measures, and overall wellness. This awareness contributes to improved health outcomes and, consequently, increased longevity. On the other hand, limited education may result in a lack of awareness about healthcare planning, potentially leading to inadequate health protection and impacting overall longevity.

The intricate relationship between effective retirement planning and longevity is a multifaceted aspect of financial well-being. Examining this connection entails delving into how individuals' readiness for retirement, the financial decisions made during this period, and the overall financial security in this life stage can influence their longevity. Individuals engaging in effective retirement planning tend to focus on building long-term financial security. This includes strategies such as consistent saving, investments, and minimising debt during their working years.

Engaging in early planning aids individuals in mitigating the financial stress associated with retirement. Reduced stress levels are correlated with improved mental and physical health, potentially contributing to an extended lifespan. Retirees who are well-prepared often demonstrate elevated financial literacy, enabling them to make informed decisions about managing their pension, Social Security benefits, and other sources of income.

Individuals with financial literacy are less prone to succumbing to common retirement pitfalls, such as overspending or engaging in risky investments, which can have implications for financial stability and longevity. Sound retirement planning encompasses the diversification of income sources, including pensions, savings, investments, and Social Security.

Diversification serves as a safety net against economic fluctuations and bolsters financial resilience. Those heavily reliant on Social Security may encounter challenges in upholding their desired standard of living in retirement, potentially impacting both financial and overall well-being.

Inclusive retirement planning frequently incorporates provisions for healthcare costs. Retirees with carefully crafted plans may enjoy enhanced access to quality healthcare, positively impacting their health and longevity. Comprehensive planning may encompass factors like long-term care insurance and other provisions to address potential health-related expenses, thereby mitigating the impact on financial resources.

Retirees who strategically plan for social engagement and community involvement may encounter enhanced mental health and a heightened sense of purpose, factors linked to increased longevity.

Those who are financially secure in retirement may possess the means to sustain healthier lifestyles, incorporating regular physical activity, a balanced diet, and access to recreational activities, all contributing to overall well-being. Retirees with effective planning are also more inclined to adapt to economic changes, such as market fluctuations or unexpected expenses, without jeopardising their financial security.

Retirees endowed with financial flexibility can tailor their lifestyle, travel plans, or housing arrangements as necessary, fostering a stress-free retirement and potentially promoting longevity. Strategic retirement planning frequently includes considerations for estate planning, encompassing the thoughtful distribution of assets to heirs.

Legacy planning, in turn, may contribute to a sense of purpose and familial well-being. Retirees who have meticulously planned for retirement often encounter heightened satisfaction and fulfilment during this life stage. Contentment is intricately linked to positive mental health and overall longevity.

The ability to financially support a healthy lifestyle, encompassing a balanced diet and regular physical activity, is crucial in shaping post-retirement health outcomes. Investigating how retirees allocate funds for recreational activities and hobbies provides insights into their capacity to maintain an active and engaged lifestyle, influencing both physical and mental health.

Retirees who are financially stable are more apt to afford suitable and comfortable living arrangements, thereby influencing their overall well-being and potentially mitigating stress-related health issues.

Examining the impact of economic downturns on public health and life expectancy yields a comprehensive understanding of the sophisticated relationship between economic stability and overall well-being. Economic downturns frequently lead to diminished healthcare accessibility, attributed to job losses and a decline in employer-sponsored health insurance. Individuals may defer or forego essential medical care due to financial constraints.

Financial constraints during economic downturns might curtail investments in preventive healthcare services, potentially resulting in a rise in preventable diseases and affecting life expectancy. Economic recessions can contribute to increased stress, anxiety, and depression due to factors such as unemployment, financial strain, and uncertainty.

Mental health challenges have the potential to adversely impact overall well-being and life expectancy. Investigating how economic downturns impact access to mental health services sheds light on the potential consequences for mental health outcomes and life expectancy.

Economic contractions may trigger job losses and income reductions, resulting in elevated levels of food insecurity. Economic downturns can instigate alterations in dietary patterns, potentially culminating in an uptick in chronic diseases linked to poor nutrition, such as obesity and cardiovascular issues.

Economic stressors may also contribute to an increase in substance abuse and addiction. The intersection between mental health challenges during economic downturns and the potential rise in substance abuse can have significant implications for public health outcomes.

Economic downturns frequently coincide with housing challenges and homelessness. Economic contractions may exacerbate educational inequalities, influencing long-term health outcomes. Economic hardships can strain social support networks and community cohesion.

Vulnerable populations, including low-income communities, may face exacerbated challenges during economic downturns. Economic downturns may exacerbate technological disparities in healthcare access.

The burden of financial stress can exert a substantial impact on both mental and physical health. Persistent worries about financial stability, debt, and meeting basic needs may foster chronic anxiety. Financial stress is frequently associated with feelings of hopelessness and helplessness, contributing to the onset, or worsening of depression.

Concerns about finances can also disrupt sleep patterns, causing difficulties in falling asleep or maintaining sleep. Insufficient and disrupted sleep can lead to fatigue and a diminished ability to cope with stressors.

Long-term stress, encompassing financial stress, has been associated with an elevated risk of cardiovascular diseases, including heart attacks and hypertension. Prolonged stress has the potential to weaken the immune system, rendering individuals more vulnerable to illnesses.

Financial stress may strain relationships, leading to heightened tension, arguments, and conflicts related to financial matters. Individuals undergoing financial stress might withdraw from social activities due to feelings of embarrassment or inadequacy.

In response to financial stress, some individuals may turn to unhealthy coping mechanisms, such as substance abuse or overeating. The impact of financial stress extends to the workplace, causing reduced concentration and productivity. The fear of job loss or unemployment can contribute to stress, adversely affecting mental well-being.

Financial stress has the potential to impair cognitive function, resulting in challenges with decision-making, problem-solving, and concentration. Additionally, financial constraints may restrict access to healthcare services, hindering individuals from seeking timely medical attention and preventive care.

Navigating financial stress involves a blend of practical strategies, emotional support, and lifestyle adjustments. Develop a realistic budget to effectively manage income and expenses. Prioritise essential expenditures and pinpoint areas where spending can be curtailed.

Create and contribute to an emergency fund to serve as a financial buffer for unforeseen expenses. Seek guidance from financial advisors or credit counsellors to explore options for debt management and enhance overall financial stability.

Facilitate open communication with family members or partners regarding financial challenges, fostering a sense of shared responsibility and support. Break down financial goals into smaller, achievable steps to alleviate feelings of overwhelm. Explore part-time or freelance opportunities to supplement income.

Incorporate stress-reduction techniques like mindfulness, meditation, or deep breathing exercises into your routine. If necessary, consider seeking professional mental health support, such as therapy or counselling. Share your concerns with friends, family, or support groups as social support can offer emotional relief and practical advice.

Elevate financial literacy by participating in workshops or utilising online resources to gain a better understanding of money management. Initiate contact with creditors to discuss payment plans or negotiate interest rates, as many financial institutions may be willing to collaborate with individuals facing difficulties. Explore possibilities for career advancement, additional training, or education to enhance job security and income potential.

Explore available local community resources, including food banks, utility assistance programs, and non-profit organisations, which may extend support. Assess eligibility for government assistance programs that can provide temporary relief. Participate in long-term financial planning to establish clear financial goals and progress towards financial security. The existence and efficacy of social safety nets, encompassing unemployment benefits, welfare programs, and healthcare services, offer a crucial financial cushion during difficult periods.

The existence of robust social networks, encompassing family and friends, serves as a source of both emotional and financial aid during challenging periods. Conversely, the absence of social support can compound financial difficulties. Cultural perspectives on money, savings, and expenditures play a significant role in shaping individual financial habits. Societal norms and expectations can impact choices concerning debt, investment, and financial planning.

Government policies, encompassing taxation, social programs, and economic regulations, wield substantial influence over income distribution, job prospects, and the overall economic landscape, thereby shaping financial well-being at a societal level. The accessibility of technology and financial services, spanning banking, investment platforms, and online resources, can impact individuals' capacity to manage their finances effectively.

The prevailing economic environment, inclusive of factors like inflation rates, interest rates, and overall stability, plays a pivotal role in determining employment opportunities, income levels, and the cost of living.

Effectively addressing socioeconomic determinants necessitates a holistic strategy involving diverse policies and programs focused on enhancing the social, economic, and health conditions of individuals and communities. Investing in high-quality early childhood education serves as a vital step in levelling the playing field for children from various socioeconomic backgrounds.

Ensuring an equitable distribution of resources and funding to schools contributes to diminishing educational disparities. The establishment and periodic adjustment of minimum wage levels play a crucial role in guaranteeing that workers receive a fair income. Government-sponsored programs designed to offer training and support can prove instrumental for individuals seeking employment or aiming for career advancement.

Implementing tax credits for low-income individuals and families can serve as a valuable supplement to their income. Advocate for initiatives that facilitate access to banking services, particularly in underserved communities. Introduce programs dedicated to enhancing financial literacy, empowering individuals to make well-informed financial decisions.

Collaborative efforts between government initiatives and private-sector partnerships to invest in infrastructure, affordable housing, and economic development within disadvantaged communities are necessary. Establish programs that offer funding, training, and resources to support the growth of small businesses, with a particular focus on underserved areas.

Financial incentives wield substantial influence over health-related choices and decision-making. Individuals frequently assess the costs and benefits of various health behaviours and leveraging financial incentives can serve as a potent means to promote positive behaviours or discourage detrimental ones.

Certain health insurance plans incorporate premium discounts or reduced deductibles for individuals actively participating in wellness programs or meeting specific health-related criteria. Waiving co-pays or deductibles for preventive services, such as vaccinations or screenings, can effectively motivate individuals to adopt proactive health behaviours.

Employers often extend financial incentives, such as bonuses or lowered health insurance premiums, to employees actively engaging in workplace wellness programs. Some employers go further by offering subsidies or reimbursements for gym memberships and fitness-related expenses to promote physical activity.

Governments, on the other hand, may introduce tax credits for designated health-related expenses, encouraging the adoption of healthier lifestyles and investment in preventive care. Additionally, levying taxes on unhealthy products like sugary beverages or tobacco serves as a deterrent, dissuading individuals from partaking in these behaviours.

Health insurance plans or pharmacy benefit programs frequently feature reduced co-pays for generic medications, motivating individuals to opt for cost-effective options. In some cases, plans introduce financial incentives for those who diligently adhere to prescribed medication regimens, leading to improved overall health outcomes. To encourage healthier choices, individuals may receive cash rewards or enjoy reduced insurance premiums for successfully quitting smoking or achieving specific health-related goals.

In the realm of community well-being, financial incentives can be intricately linked to the pursuit of collective health goals. Collaborative efforts between employers and local communities to champion health initiatives are manifesting in the form of enticing financial rewards for active participation.

Premium discounts may be linked to participating in biometric screenings and achieving specific health metrics. Financial incentives may be offered to patients who actively engage in remote monitoring programs, promoting better management of chronic conditions. Incentives can be tied to adherence to prescribed treatment plans, ensuring better health outcomes.

Motivate individuals to dedicate themselves to their health objectives by employing contracts or public commitments. For instance, the act of signing a commitment to engage in regular exercise or quit smoking has been shown to enhance adherence.

Acknowledging the prevalent tendency to prioritise immediate rewards over long-term benefits, interventions can incorporate immediate positive feedback for healthy choices or set shorter-term goals. Visual and environmental cues play a pivotal role in triggering healthier behaviours, for instance, strategically placing signs promoting stair use near elevators can effectively prompt individuals to opt for a more active alternative.

Integrate elements reminiscent of gaming, such as rewards, competition, and progress tracking, into the pursuit of healthier lifestyles to enhance engagement and enjoyment. Framing health information in a positive context tends to be more persuasive; for instance, highlighting the advantages of a healthy diet rather than the risks of an unhealthy one. Enhance the convenience of making healthy choices by minimising obstacles, whether it's strategically placing bike racks near entrances or ensuring that wholesome snacks are easily accessible.

The complex relationship between finances and longevity cannot be overstated. As we navigate the complexities of life, economic well-being emerges as a significant determinant of our ability to access quality healthcare, maintain a nourishing lifestyle, and secure the resources necessary for a prolonged and fulfilling existence.

The impact of financial stability on longevity extends beyond mere monetary considerations, reaching into the realms of mental and physical well-being. Recognising and addressing the socioeconomic factors that influence longevity is paramount, as it opens avenues for creating a more equitable and healthier future for all. In the symphony of factors shaping our lifespans, the notes of financial stability play a crucial melody, influencing the rhythm and harmony of our collective well-being.

Chapter 12 – The Impact of Religion on Longevity

The impact of religion on longevity is a compelling and intricate subject that delves into the interconnected realms of spirituality, health, and human well-being. Across diverse cultures and societies, religious beliefs and practices have been associated with various influences on the length and quality of life.

The relationship between religious engagement and longevity encompasses a spectrum of factors, ranging from lifestyle choices and social support networks to the profound psychological and emotional effects of spiritual practices.

Understanding how religious affiliations and activities contribute to an individual's lifespan involves a nuanced exploration of the intricate ways in which faith intersects with physical, mental, and social dimensions of health. This exploration sheds light on the profound and multifaceted impact that religious beliefs can have on the human journey toward a longer and more fulfilling existence.

Religious convictions wield a profound impact on the decisions individuals make in their day-to-day lives, significantly shaping their dietary preferences, exercise regimens, and perspectives on substance use. Numerous religious traditions provide explicit guidelines governing food intake, with dietary restrictions and practices deeply entrenched in cultural and spiritual principles.

Take, for instance, certain faiths that champion vegetarianism or place constraints on the consumption of types of meat. In doing so, these dietary choices become intertwined with spiritual values, reflecting the intricate intersection of religious beliefs and lifestyle preferences.

In the realm of religious teachings, there is a recurrent emphasis on regarding the body as a sacred vessel, urging followers to actively participate in regular physical activities and place a paramount focus on their overall well-being. Numerous faiths dissuade or outright forbid the consumption of substances like alcohol, tobacco, or recreational drugs.

This advocacy shapes a lifestyle ethos that prioritises health and abstains from potentially detrimental behaviours. By exerting influence over these fundamental facets of daily life, religious beliefs weave a substantial contribution into the intricate fabric of individual health, thereby influencing the potential for extended longevity.

The significance of religious practices extends beyond the spiritual realm, playing a pivotal role in delivering emotional support, mitigating stress, and cultivating mental well-being. This collective impact contributes to the prospect of a more extended and healthier life.

The communal and ritualistic dimensions inherent in religious engagement establish a structured framework, that aids individuals in effectively navigating the myriad challenges encountered on life's journey.

Engaging with religious communities frequently imparts a profound sense of belonging and fosters a supportive social network. The shared values, beliefs, and collective experiences within these communities form the bedrock for emotional support, particularly during challenging periods.

Whether manifested through communal prayers, fellowship, or participation in religious ceremonies, individuals discover solace and empathy among their peers. This shared connection serves to alleviate emotional burdens and fortify psychological resilience.

Religious practices often integrate meditative and contemplative elements, exemplified by activities like prayer or mindfulness exercises. Participation in these practices extends a calming influence on both the mind and body, effectively diminishing stress levels.

The structured design of religious rituals plays a crucial role by instilling a sense of order and purpose, providing a sanctuary from the tumultuous nature of everyday life. This structured framework emerges as a valuable coping mechanism during moments of heightened stress.

In the realm of religious teachings, there is a consistent emphasis on values like compassion, forgiveness, and gratitude, all of which work to foster positive mental attitudes. The sense of purpose and meaning derived from steadfast adherence to these religious principles contributes significantly to cultivating a more optimistic outlook on life.

Furthermore, religious communities frequently extend their support by offering counselling and pastoral care services, creating a nurturing environment for individuals contending with mental health challenges.

Religious beliefs offer a structured framework for comprehending and navigating life's uncertainties, encompassing moments of illness, loss, and existential contemplation. Whether anchored in the belief in a higher power, a divine purpose, or the interconnectedness of all things, these convictions provide individuals with a coping mechanism that surpasses immediate challenges. This cultivated resilience and coping capacity wields a positive influence on mental well-being and, consequently, contribute to the broader spectrum of overall health.

Through tending to emotional needs, alleviating stress, and nurturing mental well-being, religious practices contribute to a comprehensive approach to health that transcends mere physical dimensions. The symbiotic relationship between emotional and mental health and the prospect of an extended life underscores the pivotal role that religious engagement can play in fostering overall well-being.

The communal facets of religious involvement encompass the shared experiences, connections, and social networks forged within religious communities. Religious gatherings, services, and events offer occasions for individuals to unite, cultivating a profound sense of belonging and shared identity. This communal engagement frequently transcends formal religious undertakings, permeating diverse facets of individuals' lives.

Religious communities provide a haven where individuals sharing similar beliefs and values unite, fostering a profound sense of belonging and shared identity. This connection and shared purpose form the bedrock of a resilient social support network.

Engaging in religious communities not only forges social networks characterised by mutual care and support but also cultivates connections grounded in common values, beliefs, and goals. These robust social ties extend beyond the confines of religious institutions, permeating various facets of individuals' personal and social lives.

Religious communities consistently underscore the significance of mutual care. Within these congregations, members actively participate in acts of kindness, offer emotional support, and extend help during times of adversity. These nurturing relationships wield positive impacts on mental health, contributing significantly to overall well-being.

Shared ethical and moral frameworks prevalent in religious societies guide behaviour. This collective set of values nurtures trust and cooperation among members, establishing a supportive environment where individuals can confidently depend on one another for assistance, guidance, and encouragement.

Consistent engagement in religious rituals, ceremonies, and celebrations serves to deepen social bonds within the community. These communal activities offer moments of shared joy, gratitude, and a profound sense of unity, thereby fortifying the social fabric that contributes to overall well-being. The implications of these communal aspects on health outcomes and lifespan can be notably impactful.

Strong social support networks have been linked to an array of health advantages, encompassing reduced levels of stress, depression, and chronic diseases. The emotional and practical support cultivated within religious communities plays a pivotal role in fostering improved mental health and effective coping mechanisms during challenging circumstances. Individuals with robust social ties, often nurtured within religious groups, may encounter enhanced health and an extended lifespan.

Religious beliefs and practices frequently emerge as potent coping mechanisms amid life's challenges, illnesses, or losses. These coping strategies delve into the spiritual and psychological dimensions of an individual's worldview, furnishing a structured approach to comprehend and traverse trying circumstances. Religious beliefs construct a framework for grasping the meaning and purpose embedded in life's trials.

In these convictions, individuals discover solace, finding reassurance in the notion of a higher purpose or divine plan that imparts significance even during adversity. This imbued sense of purpose correlates with positive mental health outcomes and holds the potential to contribute to overall well-being.

Rituals like prayer and meditation constitute prevalent elements in religious traditions. Participation in these activities facilitates a connection to something greater, extending comfort and a channel for contemplation. Prayer can be linked to diminished stress levels and enhanced emotional well-being, suggesting potential effects on physical health.

In times of adversity, illness, or loss, religious communities frequently unite to support individuals. The communal backing from fellow believers becomes a pivotal facet of coping. The emotional and practical support bestowed by a religious community may diminish feelings of isolation and nurture resilience.

The rituals and ceremonies inherent in religious practices offer individuals structured avenues for processing and expressing their emotions. These ceremonial acts can function as symbolic avenues of healing, signifying transitions, and bestowing a sense of closure. Active participation in religious ceremonies may yield positive effects on mental health and contribute to the healing journey during times of grief.

Religious beliefs often centre around themes of hope, resilience, and the potential for transcendence. The belief in a higher power or a guiding force has the capacity to instil a profound sense of hope, a factor associated with improved mental health outcomes and an enhanced ability to navigate stress.

Numerous religious traditions underscore the significance of forgiveness and compassion, even in the face of adversity. The act of forgiveness, when practiced, holds the potential to foster emotional healing, diminish resentment, and nurture positive mental health, thereby exerting an influence on overall well-being.

In the pursuit of healing, some individuals weave spiritual practices, such as prayer, meditation, or other rituals, into their therapeutic journey, considering them complementary to medical treatments.

Adopting this integrated perspective enhances our grasp of health and recovery. Participation in religious practices is associated with reduced levels of anxiety and stress. The rituals, routines, and spiritual guidance woven into religious beliefs function as protective shields against the psychological and physiological tolls of stress, potentially exerting an impact on overall health.

Religious affiliations exert influence on healthcare access through a network of interconnected factors, encompassing healthcare-seeking behaviours, trust in medical institutions, and adherence to medical advice. The interplay of these dynamics is sculpted by cultural, social, and personal beliefs intertwined with one's religious identity.

Religious beliefs play a role in determining whether individuals adopt proactive or reactive healthcare-seeking behaviours. Certain religious communities may prioritise preventive care and regular check-ups, whereas others may place greater reliance on faith-based healing practices, thereby influencing the timing and frequency of seeking medical attention.

Specific religious groups might favour or depend on alternative medicine practices in alignment with their beliefs, thereby influencing the healthcare they pursue. This inclination can lead to variations in decisions related to traditional medical treatments, resulting in diverse patterns of healthcare utilisation.

The level of trust in medical institutions can be influenced by the cultural competence of healthcare providers. Individuals with religious affiliations may find greater comfort in seeking care from providers who comprehend and respect their religious beliefs, consequently shaping trust levels and willingness to engage in healthcare interactions.

The perceived religious affiliation of healthcare institutions plays a significant role in shaping trust dynamics. Individuals may find greater comfort seeking care from institutions aligned with their religious beliefs, while conversely, reservations may arise if a perceived lack of alignment exists.

Religious beliefs extend their influence on treatment choices, impacting adherence to medical advice. For instance, specific faith traditions may highlight prayer and spiritual practices as integral components of healing, thereby influencing the acceptance or rejection of medical interventions.

Certain religious communities might espouse fatalistic perspectives, attributing health outcomes to divine will. Such views can impact adherence to medical advice, as individuals may be less inclined to actively engage in proactive health management if they believe outcomes are predestined.

Cultural norms within religious communities play a role in influencing adherence to medical advice. Stigma surrounding specific health conditions or treatments may instil reluctance in following medical recommendations, consequently influencing health outcomes.

Religious communities frequently function as vital social support networks, exerting an influence on the accessibility of healthcare resources. The existence of healthcare facilities affiliated with a particular religion or community-based health initiative can significantly improve accessibility for members of specific religious groups.

Economic considerations within religious communities may also shape healthcare access. Some religious groups might prioritise community-based financial support for healthcare needs, while others could encounter barriers arising from economic disparities.

The influence of religious affiliations on healthcare access is intricate and multifaceted. Grasping these dynamics is imperative for healthcare providers, enabling the delivery of culturally competent care that honours and accommodates individuals' religious beliefs. This approach not only fosters better health outcomes but also cultivates increased trust in medical institutions within diverse communities.

Religious beliefs wield a profound influence, endowing individuals with a sense of purpose, meaning, and direction in life. This influence, in turn, carries significant implications for mental and emotional well-being, potentially contributing to longevity.

Within the realm of religious beliefs lies a set of guiding principles, moral values, and a sense of purpose derived from allegiance to a higher power or divine plan. This framework not only imparts a clear understanding of an individual's purpose in life but also bestows a profound sense of meaning that extends beyond individual experiences.

Numerous religious teachings underscore the notion of transcending individual desires and self-interest, encouraging a concentration on contributing to the well-being of others and the broader community. This altruistic perspective fosters a profound sense of purpose that goes beyond personal achievements. In moments of adversity, like illness, loss, or life challenges, religious beliefs often emerge as potent coping mechanisms. The belief in a higher power, divine plan, or ultimate purpose serves as a source of comfort, solace, and resilience, acting as a buffer against stress and emotional distress.

Individuals with religious affiliations often express elevated levels of hope and optimism. The belief in a greater purpose to life and the understanding that challenges are integral to a broader plan cultivates a positive outlook, fostering emotional well-being and mental resilience in challenging situations.

Religious communities frequently function as wellsprings of social support. Shared beliefs and values forge robust social bonds that provide emotional assistance during adversity. This communal support contributes significantly to a sense of belonging, diminishing feelings of isolation and loneliness.

The coping mechanisms inherent in religious beliefs, encompassing practices like prayer, meditation, and finding solace in faith, have been correlated with lower stress levels. Given that chronic stress is a recognised contributor to various health issues, the alleviation of stress through religious practices may play a role in promoting overall well-being and potentially contributing to increased longevity.

The sense of purpose stemming from religious beliefs holds sway over lifestyle choices. Individuals with a well-defined purpose are often more predisposed to embrace healthier behaviours, encompassing regular exercise, balanced diets, and abstention from harmful substances, factors that contribute to an extended life expectancy.

The emotional resilience fostered by religious beliefs can wield a positive influence on health outcomes. Individuals with robust religious or spiritual beliefs tend to exhibit enhanced resilience in the face of health challenges, potentially influencing both recovery and longevity.

Religious beliefs afford individuals a profound sense of purpose, meaning, and direction in life, nurturing mental and emotional well-being. The coping mechanisms drawn from faith play a role in bolstering emotional resilience, reducing stress, and fostering a positive outlook. These elements, coupled with potential impacts on lifestyle choices, might contribute to an extended lifespan among individuals with robust religious affiliations.

Religious traditions and cultural practices affiliated with distinct faiths exert substantial influence on lifestyle factors that profoundly affect health. Particularly, dietary restrictions and cleanliness rituals emerge as pivotal elements shaping the well-being of individuals within these religious communities.

Numerous religious traditions prescribe explicit dietary guidelines, delineating permissible and prohibited foods. These restrictions typically find their roots in spiritual beliefs and cultural practices. For example, certain faiths endorse vegetarianism, while others may have regulations regarding the consumption of specific meats or the observance of fasting periods.

Adhering to religious dietary restrictions holds sway over nutritional intake and dietary habits, potentially leading to diets abundant in specific nutrients that can impact health outcomes. Conversely, the strict limitations imposed by religious dietary practices may demand careful consideration to ensure individuals meet their nutritional needs.

Many religious traditions integrate rituals linked to cleanliness and purification. These practices, including ablution or ceremonial cleansing, carry symbolic and spiritual significance. Furthermore, cleanliness rituals often extend to the home environment, underscoring the importance of maintaining a tidy and sanctified living space.

The prioritisation of cleanliness in religious rituals can manifest tangible effects on health. Consistent cleansing practices actively contribute to personal hygiene, diminishing the risk of infections and fostering overall well-being. Furthermore, the dedication to maintaining a clean and orderly environment is linked to psychological benefits and stress reduction.

In religious communities, the communal bonds formed often create tight-knit social networks where cultural practices related to health are shared and reinforced. For instance, communal gatherings may involve specific dietary choices or cleanliness rituals.

The shared commitment to cleanliness practices within the community fosters a supportive environment that encourages health-conscious behaviours. The infusion of religious and cultural values into everyday life extends to broader lifestyle choices, encompassing decisions regarding physical activity, sleep patterns, and stress management. The synchronisation of these choices with religious teachings contributes to a comprehensive approach to health within the framework of cultural and spiritual practices.

The influence of religion on longevity is a sophisticated phenomenon intricately interwoven into the tapestry of individuals' lives, communities, and societal structures. Religious beliefs wield a profound influence on various dimensions of well-being, spanning physical, mental, and emotional aspects. The pathways through which religion may contribute to longevity are diverse and interconnected, unveiling a complex interplay of factors.

Recognising the diversity within religious traditions and the dynamic nature of the connection between religion and longevity is essential. Disparities exist not only among different faiths but also within specific religious groups, highlighting the influence of cultural, regional, and individual factors. The impact of religion on longevity is not a uniform phenomenon, ongoing research delves into the nuanced intersections between diverse religious beliefs and health outcomes.

As we navigate this complex landscape, it becomes evident that understanding the role of religion in longevity requires a holistic perspective, one that considers the rich tapestry of beliefs, practices, and cultural contexts within which individuals live their lives. Acknowledging these complexities provides a foundation for fostering culturally competent healthcare, supporting diverse communities in their pursuit of well-being, and appreciating the multifaceted nature of the human experience.

Ultimately, the impact of religion on longevity represents a dynamic and evolving field of study, inviting continued exploration and dialogue at the intersection of faith, health, and the human journey toward a longer and more fulfilling life.

Chapter 13 - Blue Zones and Longevity Hotspots

In various corners of the globe, there exist enclaves known as Blue Zones, where inhabitants seem to defy the conventional expectations of ageing. Within these realms, individuals not only enjoy extended lifespans but also experience a remarkable state of health that sets them apart from the global norm. These locales have become focal points of interest due to their elevated numbers of centenarians, those who gracefully cross the threshold of one hundred years, and the notable scarcity of age-related ailments.

Within each Blue Zone, a distinctive tapestry of cultural nuances, dietary practices, and lifestyles weaves together to foster the extraordinary longevity witnessed among its residents. Shared among these diverse locales are recurring threads, commitment to a plant-centric diet, a regimen of regular physical activity, robust social bonds, a sense of purpose, and an ethos of low-stress living.

The emergence of Blue Zones has kindled a burgeoning curiosity about the parallels that unite these regions and the potential application of their guiding principles to cultivate healthier and lengthier lives in disparate communities. Worldwide, researchers and health enthusiasts are engrossed in dissecting the intricacies of Blue Zones, endeavouring to distil valuable lessons on longevity and overall well-being.

At the core of the Blue Zones concept lies the belief that specific lifestyle, dietary, and social elements play pivotal roles in enhancing both longevity and overall well-being. Rigorous research and meticulous analysis have unveiled shared characteristics and practices within various Blue Zones, offering profound insights into the factors that contribute to a life that is both long and healthy.

Inhabitants of Blue Zones frequently adhere to a primarily plant-based diet, embracing the abundance of fruits, vegetables, whole grains, and legumes. The intake of meat is generally modest, reflecting a dietary pattern focused on plant-derived foods. Engaging in daily physical activity is a prevalent norm within Blue Zones, with an emphasis on activities like walking, gardening, or other forms of moderate physical exertion, eschewing the need for intense workouts.

Beyond dietary and exercise practices, the social fabric of Blue Zones is woven with threads of strong interpersonal connections and active community participation. The significance of supportive social networks and a profound sense of belonging cannot be overstated, playing pivotal roles in mitigating stress levels, and fostering heightened overall well-being.

A shared characteristic among Blue Zone inhabitants is the possession of a distinct sense of purpose in life. This purpose, whether rooted in cultural, religious, or personal beliefs, serves as a compelling motivation for individuals to rise each morning and actively engage in their pursuits. Notably, the populations in Blue Zones commonly exercise moderation in their dietary habits, avoiding overindulgence. This practice aligns with the longevity-enhancing benefits associated with calorie restriction.

Additionally, Blue Zone communities exhibit lower levels of chronic stress, a phenomenon attributed to several contributing factors. The presence of robust social support networks, the incorporation of regular physical activity into daily life, and an overarching emphasis on maintaining a positive mindset collectively contribute to the stress-reducing environment within these populations.

Ikaria, nestled in the Aegean Sea, stands as a Greek island celebrated for its remarkable proportion of centenarians. Renowned for their adherence to the Mediterranean diet, the inhabitants of Ikaria epitomise an active lifestyle, robust social bonds, and a serene pace of life. On the other side of the globe, Okinawa, a Japanese island, boasts one of the world's highest life expectancies. The Okinawan way of life centres around a plant-based diet, routine physical activity, and a profound sense of purpose encapsulated by the concept of "ikigai."

In the mountainous expanse of Barbagia in Sardinia, Italy, a notable prevalence of centenarians has garnered attention. Rooted in the Sardinian way of life, characterised by a diet rich in whole foods and fortified by resilient family and community ties, longevity flourishes in this region.

Venturing to the Nicoya Peninsula in Costa Rica unveils another enclave of exceptional longevity. Here, centenarians abound, their diet anchored in staples like beans, corn, and squash. Augmenting their dietary choices are the twin pillars of a robust sense of community and a leisurely pace of life, both contributing to the remarkable longevity witnessed in this region.

In the case of Loma Linda, California, USA, a distinctive facet of the Blue Zones emerges, it's not a specific geographic area but a community. This community is home to a group of Seventh-day Adventists who adhere to a vegetarian diet, engage in regular physical activity, and prioritise both rest and spiritual practices. In this unique Blue Zone, the synthesis of lifestyle choices within a close-knit community fosters an environment conducive to enhanced well-being and longevity.

Delving into the lifestyle practices common among Blue Zone residents has brought to light discernible patterns deemed instrumental in their extraordinary longevity and well-being. While the particulars may exhibit variation across different Blue Zones, overarching themes permeate the lifestyles of these diverse populations.

A pivotal element in Blue Zones is the prevalent adoption of a predominantly plant-based diet. Inhabitants of these regions embrace a diverse array of fruits, vegetables, whole grains, legumes, and nuts in their daily culinary choices. Additionally, a characteristic trait of Blue Zone populations is their practice of moderation in food consumption, eschewing overindulgence and, to some extent, incorporating calorie restriction.

Concurrent with dietary practices is the routine engagement in regular, low-intensity physical activity, a habitual norm within Blue Zones. Activities such as walking, gardening, and other forms of moderate exercise seamlessly integrate into the daily rhythms of these communities.

Inhabitants of Blue Zones seamlessly incorporate physical activities into their daily routines, whether it be walking to work or attending to their agricultural endeavours. The adoption of formal exercise regimens is less prevalent within these communities. One of the unifying factors across Blue Zones is the presence of positive social interactions and robust community bonds.

The intertwined elements of social support and a profound sense of belonging play integral roles in mitigating stress levels and nurturing overall well-being. Within the Blue Zone ethos, there exists a pronounced emphasis on close-knit family relationships. Often, multiple generations cohabit in proximity, fostering a tangible sense of connection and mutual support that contributes to the distinctive fabric of these communities.

In the tranquil landscapes of Okinawa, the essence of ikigai and the profound philosophy of "Panta Rei" in Ikaria converge, embodying a deep-rooted purpose and significance in one's existence. The understanding that a compelling reason to greet each dawn is fundamental for a long and fulfilling life resonates harmoniously across the Blue Zones. Inhabitants of these longevity-centric regions consistently express diminished levels of persistent stress, a consequence of robust social networks, close-knit community ties, and an optimistic perspective towards life.

Furthermore, within specific Blue Zones, an embrace of spiritual or religious practices stands as a prevailing norm. This entails regular attendance at religious gatherings and active engagement in communal rituals, serving as additional pillars of strength for the holistic well-being of these extraordinary communities.

A measured intake of alcohol is a prevalent practice, with a preference for local and traditional libations consumed judiciously. Actively engaging in community events and rituals is a recurring theme, as inhabitants of Blue Zones actively contribute to the communal fabric, fostering a profound sense of purpose and connection.

It's crucial to acknowledge that while these behavioural patterns offer valuable insights, individual diversities and cultural subtleties are inherent within each Blue Zone. Recognising the adaptability of these principles to various cultures and communities becomes imperative for the widespread promotion of healthier lifestyles globally.

Blue Zones consistently prioritise plant-based nutrition, with diets featuring an abundance of fruits, vegetables, whole grains, legumes, and nuts. The prevalence of the Mediterranean diet is notable, emphasising the consumption of olive oil and fish while limiting red meat intake. Residents of Blue Zones adopt a balanced approach to their dietary habits, exercising moderation in food consumption.

A prevalent theme in Blue Zone nutrition is caloric restriction, strategically implemented to extend longevity and lower the risk of age-related diseases, all without compromising essential nutritional needs. Furthermore, these diets often revolve around locally sourced and seasonal foods, fostering sustainable agricultural practices. This approach not only contributes to environmental well-being but also ensures a diverse and nutrient-rich dietary intake for the residents.

Meals in Blue Zones are frequently enjoyed in the company of family and friends, underscoring the social dimension of eating. This communal approach to dining fosters a positive connection with food, elevating the overall gastronomic experience. Residents of Blue Zones integrate regular, low-intensity physical activities seamlessly into their daily routines.

Everyday pursuits such as walking, gardening, and manual labour are woven into the fabric of their lifestyles. Formal exercise isn't necessarily a regimented part of their daily schedule. Instead, physical activity is naturally incorporated into their lives, be it walking to work, tending to gardens, or participating in traditional dances. This organic integration of movement into daily life aligns with the Blue Zone philosophy, contributing to the holistic well-being of its inhabitants.

In Blue Zones, physical activities predominantly centre around functional fitness, aimed at preserving individuals' capacity to carry out daily tasks as they age. The prevalent practice of walking or biking for transportation serves a dual purpose, not only does it encourage physical activity, but it also diminishes dependence on motorised vehicles.

Within Blue Zone communities, there is a concerted emphasis on nurturing social connections. Cultivating positive relationships with family, friends, and neighbours plays a pivotal role in enhancing emotional well-being and fostering resilience. Engaging actively in community events and rituals serves as a powerful catalyst for fortifying social bonds.

This active participation cultivates a profound sense of belonging and a shared purpose among individuals. Many Blue Zone societies embrace the concept of multigenerational living, with several generations cohabiting in proximity. This arrangement facilitates frequent interactions and mutual support among family members.

The inclusion of traditional cultural rituals and ceremonies offers valuable opportunities for socialising and reinforcing a collective identity. These events play a pivotal role in nurturing a sense of community and fostering meaningful connections. While technology is not entirely absent, Blue Zone communities often prioritise face-to-face communication over virtual interactions, leading to the cultivation of deeper and more meaningful connections.

Delving into the intricacies of the communities nestled within the enigmatic Blue Zones unveils an embroidery of distinctive traits and cultural rituals that underpin the remarkable longevity and flourishing health witnessed in these locales. In Ikaria, a beacon of such longevity, the embodiment of the Mediterranean diet stands out prominently.

This culinary philosophy boasts a rich repertoire of elements, from the elevated consumption of vegetables, olive oil, legumes, to the reverence for whole grains. Notably, the inclusion of fish and dairy further punctuates the dietary mosaic embraced by the denizens of Ikaria.

A prominent facet of Ikarian dietary practices involves the habitual enjoyment of herbal teas, crafted from indigenous herbs believed to harbour potential health advantages. Beyond the culinary realm, Ikarian communities are distinguished by a serene cadence of life and a profound commitment to fostering social bonds.

The convivial act of gathering in local cafes, affectionately termed "kafenia," is a widespread tradition. Amidst the undulating landscapes of Ikaria, a culture of physical engagement thrives, manifesting in the routine pursuits of walking and tending to gardens, seamlessly woven into the fabric of everyday existence.

Okinawa is renowned for its adherence to the "Okinawan diet," a culinary tapestry rich in sweet potatoes, vegetables, tofu, and seaweed. The dietary tableau also embraces the regular consumption of fish, with a conscious limitation on red meat. Beyond the realm of nutrition, the cultural essence of Okinawa is encapsulated in the concept of ikigai, a profound philosophy embodying "a reason for being" or "a reason to wake up in the morning." This ideology contributes significantly to a palpable sense of purpose among Okinawans.

Within the daily rhythm of Okinawan life, the cultivation of green tea takes centre stage, particularly the locally grown variety known as "goya tea," believed to bestow health benefits. The social fabric is interwoven with the practice of living in multigenerational households, fostering close-knit family bonds and robust support systems.

Sardinians adhere faithfully to a Mediterranean diet characterised by an abundance of fruits, vegetables, whole grains, olive oil, and measured servings of dairy and meat. Notably, the moderate consumption of local red wine, especially the renowned Cannonau wine, is knottily linked with the impressive longevity observed among the Sardinian population.

Within the enchanting realm of Barbagia, a region within Sardinia, a remarkable concentration of centenarians thrives, with specific villages like Ogliastra identified as flourishing longevity hotspots. The vibrant drapery of Sardinian life is further enriched by traditional festivals and celebrations, serving as meaningful occasions that fortify the social fabric of these communities.

At the heart of the traditional Nicoya diet lies a harmonious blend of beans, corn, and squash, artfully complemented by an array of tropical fruits and locally sourced vegetables. The water in Nicoya, renowned for its elevated calcium content, plays a pivotal role in fostering robust bone health among its inhabitants. Deeply rooted in their cultural ethos, Nicoyans prioritise and cherish familial relationships, often choosing to reside in multigenerational households.

In Nicoya, the elderly continues to play an active and meaningful role in community life, contributing not only to the collective wisdom of the society but also fostering a profound sense of purpose among its members.

Loma Linda stands apart as a distinctive community, not defined by geographical boundaries but rather by its affiliation with Seventh-day Adventists who frequently adopt a vegetarian diet. Central to their way of life is the observance of the Sabbath, an essential day devoted to rest and spiritual contemplation. This dedicated time encompasses moments for family, worship, and relaxation, underscoring the integral role of spiritual well-being in their lifestyle.

Residents of Loma Linda hold health in high regard, incorporating regular exercise and embracing behaviours that promote well-being. Within this tight-knit community, the bonds forged among its members serve as a robust foundation for social support, further fortifying positive health habits among its residents.

Within the enigmatic realms of Blue Zones, the fabric of society is woven with strong familial bonds and a prevalent embrace of multigenerational living arrangements. Families, functioning as pivotal support systems, not only cultivate a profound sense of belonging but also engender a cocoon of security for individuals. Central to the ethos of Blue Zones is an ingrained respect for elders, with the older generation assuming vital roles within their communities, imparting wisdom, sharing experiences, and providing invaluable guidance.

The social textile extends beyond immediate family circles, encompassing neighbours, friends, and fellow community members. These interlaced relationships form a resilient web of support, nurturing a collective strength that defines life within Blue Zones.

In Blue Zone societies, there is a notable emphasis on cooperation and collaboration, with communities frequently pooling efforts for tasks like farming, construction, and other communal responsibilities. Traditional rituals and ceremonies play a pivotal role in reinforcing cultural identity and fostering social bonds within these communities.

Milestone occasions, including birthdays and anniversaries, are not solitary affairs but rather moments of community-wide celebration. Through these shared festivities, social connections are fortified, and a collective sense of joy permeates the community, creating a sense of interconnectedness.

Within Blue Zones, distinctive dietary traditions involvedly intertwined into the cultural heritage prevail. These culinary practices, handed down through generations, play a vital role in nurturing the collective health and well-being of the community. In certain Blue Zones, a prevalent commitment to spiritual or religious practices is evident, offering a structured foundation for meaning, purpose, and a shared sense of community. Residents of Blue Zones actively engage in a wealth of community events, festivals, and gatherings. This enthusiastic involvement not only fosters a robust sense of community identity but also instils a deep sense of pride among its members.

Communities frequently partake in joint endeavours, be it in farming, construction, or other communal initiatives. This cultivates a culture of cooperation and reciprocal assistance. The commitment to social bonds extends to offering support during periods of adversity.

Whether faced with illness, loss, or other challenges, Blue Zone communities unite to provide solace to those in distress.

Hubs like community centres, gathering spots, or market squares play a vital role as focal points for social interactions. These spaces play a crucial part in nurturing a profound sense of community and belonging.

Individuals reaching the age of one hundred and beyond in Blue Zones may harbour specific genetic factors contributing to their longevity. In Sardinia, distinct genetic markers have been pinpointed within the population, suggesting a potential influence on their remarkable longevity.

The unveiling of these markers has piqued considerable interest in the realm of genetic research. Certain regions exhibit a clustering of families with an unusually high number of centenarians, suggesting a potential hereditary component.

In Blue Zones, the availability of clean air and water emerges as a cornerstone of enhanced overall health. Environmental conditions play a pivotal role in diminishing the susceptibility to respiratory and waterborne diseases. The proximity to nature and open outdoor spaces not only fosters physical activity but also provides avenues for relaxation and stress alleviation.

Centenarians in Blue Zones frequently exhibit lower levels of chronic stress. The absence of contemporary stressors, coupled with robust social support, significantly contributes to their emotional well-being. A positive mindset, resilience, and an adaptive approach to life's challenges emerge as prevalent traits among these centenarians. These psychological attributes play a pivotal role in shaping their holistic well-being.

The physical landscape emerges as a pivotal influence in sculpting the lifestyles and well-being of communities residing in Blue Zones. Environmental factors play a definitive role in contributing to the overarching health and longevity witnessed within these regions.

Frequently, Blue Zones boast access to pristine natural settings, whether it be mountainous terrains, serene beaches, or idyllic rural landscapes. This exposure to nature correlates with heightened mental well-being, diminished stress levels, and an overarching cultivation of a positive mindset among the residents.

Blue Zones commonly enjoy the advantages of unpolluted air and water, fostering favourable effects on respiratory health and mitigating the risk of waterborne diseases. The absence of pollution significantly contributes to the creation of a healthier living environment. Many Blue Zones are distinguished by communities who frequently walk, featuring pedestrian-friendly infrastructure.

This intentional layout inspires residents to incorporate regular physical activity, primarily through walking, thereby enhancing cardiovascular health and overall fitness. Moreover, Blue Zones frequently encompass fertile land that is conducive to agriculture. This allows residents to cultivate a bounty of fresh, locally sourced produce, thereby contributing to the adoption of a plant-based diet abundant in fruits and vegetables.

Blue Zones frequently enjoy temperate climates conducive to year-round outdoor living. Residents can partake in outdoor activities, socialise in public spaces, and sustain an active lifestyle irrespective of the season. Meticulously planned public areas, ranging from town squares to community parks, offer avenues for social interaction and community involvement.

These well-designed spaces actively contribute to nurturing a profound sense of community and belonging. Moreover, Blue Zones typically boast minimal exposure to industrial pollution and other environmental stressors often prevalent in urban settings. This diminished exposure plays a pivotal role in mitigating chronic stress levels among residents.

In certain Blue Zones, adherence to traditional architectural styles and living arrangements persists. This commitment to preserving cultural and historical elements serves as a linchpin in fostering a profound sense of identity and continuity within these communities. The proximity to local farms and markets ensures a direct and immediate source of fresh, seasonal foods for residents, thereby promoting and sustaining healthy eating habits.

Furthermore, Blue Zones frequently boast lower crime rates, enhancing the overall sense of safety and security within their environs. This safe living environment plays a pivotal role in positively influencing the mental well-being of the residents.

Geographical, climatic, and ecological variables exert a profound influence on the distinctive characteristics and lifestyles of communities dwelling in Blue Zones. These factors play a pivotal role in shaping the overall well-being and longevity distinctive to these regions. In some instances, Blue Zones are situated in relatively secluded areas, historically sheltered from external influences.

This isolation serves as a potential catalyst for preserving traditional lifestyles and cultural practices. In specific Blue Zones, exemplified by Ikaria in Greece, the presence of mountainous terrain adds an additional layer to the landscape. The rugged expanse may act as a catalyst for physical activity, fostering pursuits such as walking and hiking. This engagement contributes significantly to the residents' overall fitness levels.

Blue Zones typically exhibit lower levels of industrialisation and environmental pollution. This diminished exposure to environmental stressors significantly contributes to the lower prevalence of chronic stress among residents. Striking a balance between human habitation and the preservation of natural ecosystems is a hallmark of Blue Zones, fostering a harmonious living environment.

In regions endowed with diverse ecosystems, a wealth of plant-based foods and herbs may contribute to the nutritional diversity inherent in residents' diets. Furthermore, certain Blue Zones integrate locally available herbs and plants into traditional medicinal practices, offering a potential contribution to overall health.

It's crucial to recognise that, although Blue Zones offer invaluable insights into healthy living, individual factors and cultural nuances play pivotal roles in shaping health outcomes. Continuous research endeavours persist in enhancing our understanding of the mechanisms underpinning the positive health effects observed in Blue Zone populations.

The Blue Zones concept carries substantial implications for global health, providing invaluable insights and lessons that hold the potential to enhance well-being and longevity on a global scale. Central to the Blue Zones philosophy is a proactive approach to health, emphasising lifestyle practices aimed at mitigating the risk of chronic diseases. This change in basic assumptions aligns seamlessly with the global imperative to prioritise preventive healthcare measures over reactive treatment strategies.

The prominent focus on plant-based nutrition within Blue Zones underscores the necessity for worldwide dietary guidelines that prioritise the consumption of fruits, vegetables, whole grains, and legumes. Implementing such guidelines holds the potential to alleviate the burden of diet-related diseases on a global scale.

Furthermore, the incorporation of regular, low-intensity physical activity into the daily lives of Blue Zone residents highlights the pivotal importance of advocating for physical activity on a global scale. The promotion of active living and the reduction of sedentary behaviours emerge as critical components for enhancing overall health.

Blue Zones underscore the profound influence of social connections, community engagement, and a sense of purpose on health outcomes. In shaping global health strategies, due recognition and addressing of social determinants should be integral components of the overarching well-being agenda.

The efficacy of Blue Zones is deeply rooted in culturally relevant practices. Consequently, global health initiatives ought to embrace a culturally competent approach, respecting diverse cultural norms and customising interventions accordingly.

As populations age on a global scale, the lessons derived from Blue Zones offer valuable guidance for promoting healthy ageing. Strategies emphasising the preservation of functional independence, nurturing social connections, and fostering a sense of purpose assume increasing importance in the pursuit of optimal well-being.

Blue Zones thrive in environments blessed with pristine air, water, and natural landscapes. For holistic global health initiatives, there must be a concerted focus on addressing environmental factors, advocating for clean and sustainable living spaces. This approach aims to diminish the prevalence of health risks stemming from environmental conditions.

The significance placed on stress alleviation, fostering social bonds, and cultivating a positive mental outlook within Blue Zones underscores the pivotal role of mental health in overall well-being. Consequently, global health agendas should accord due priority to the promotion and support of mental health.

The guiding principles of Blue Zones extend to health education and literacy, emphasising the empowerment of individuals with the knowledge and skills needed to make informed decisions about their well-being. Therefore, on a global scale, health initiatives should centre on equipping people with the information and capabilities necessary for navigating their health journey with wisdom and confidence.

The triumph of Blue Zones underscores the imperative to merge health-promoting principles into global public policies. Policies that advocate for walkable communities, foster healthy food environments, and build robust social infrastructures can exert a positive influence on the health of populations at large.

The Blue Zones concept not only advocates for such policies but also champions global collaboration and the dissemination of best practices. In this vein, international partnerships play a crucial role in facilitating the exchange of knowledge and strategies aimed at promoting health and longevity.

The enduring health benefits witnessed in Blue Zones emphasise the economic value inherent in investing in health promotion and disease prevention. Consequently, there is a pressing need for governments and organisations to conscientiously consider the economic impact of prioritising population health. Recognising the long-term gains associated with such investments is not just a matter of health but also a strategic economic consideration.

Though the concept of Blue Zones has earned acclaim for championing healthy lifestyles and longevity, it is not immune to challenges and critique. Blue Zones are demarcated to specific geographic regions and transplanting their principles onto diverse global populations might oversimplify intricate health dynamics.

Detractors contend that insufficient consideration is given to cultural and regional variations. What proves effective in one community may not seamlessly apply to others characterised by distinct cultural norms and lifestyles. The universal applicability of Blue Zone principles thus faces scepticism considering the elaborate interplay of health factors across diverse societies.

Investigations into Blue Zones frequently engage in observational studies, and the complexities of establishing causation pose a considerable challenge. Critics contend that ascribing longevity exclusively to lifestyle factors may oversimplify the multifaceted nature of ageing. Genetic components, socioeconomic conditions, and accessibility to healthcare also contribute significantly to longevity.

While correlations between lifestyle choices and extended life spans are evident, pinpointing direct cause-and-effect relationships proves to be a formidable task. Detractors argue that attributing longevity solely to lifestyle practices overlooks other potential influences, such as genetic predispositions and environmental factors.

Blue Zones are frequently marked by homogeneous populations exhibiting specific sociodemographic and economic conditions. Detractors propose that these factors might wield considerable influence over health outcomes and duplicating Blue Zone success could prove challenging in communities marked by greater diversity and economic disparities.

Some Blue Zones have undergone shifts in demographics, migration patterns, and lifestyle owing to modernisation. Critics contend that the initial conditions of the Blue Zones may have evolved due to demographic changes and urbanisation, thereby affecting the applicability of the model in contemporary contexts.

The widespread acceptance of the Blue Zones concept has resulted in the commercialisation and marketing of products and services promising to emulate Blue Zone success. Detractors posit that commercial interests might exploit the concept, potentially giving rise to oversimplified or deceptive health claims.

Efforts to duplicate the Blue Zones model in diverse communities have not consistently produced comparable outcomes. Critics cast doubt on the scalability and replicability of Blue Zone principles, proposing that success may hinge on distinct local factors.

Blue Zones frequently highlight longevity, though not necessarily the quality of life in later years. Critics contend that a sole emphasis on extending life might overlook the crucial aspect of fostering overall well-being, encompassing mental health, mobility, and independence.

Ethical apprehensions arise concerning the monetisation of Blue Zones and the potential exploitation of communities for research objectives. Detractors underscore the necessity for ethical considerations, including community consent and fair distribution of benefits stemming from Blue Zone research.

The Blue Zones concept strongly underscores lifestyle factors as key determinants of longevity. However, critics contend that this emphasis could potentially result in assigning individual blame for health outcomes while overlooking broader systemic issues, including healthcare access, socioeconomic disparities, and environmental factors.

The discoveries from Blue Zones have sparked numerous innovations and interventions dedicated to fostering health, well-being, and longevity. Acknowledging the challenges and critiques, the affirmative facets of Blue Zones have fuelled inventive approaches in healthcare, community development, and public health.

Urban planners are integrating Blue Zone principles into their designs, focusing on crafting walkable communities, prioritising pedestrian-friendly infrastructure, and establishing public spaces that promote physical activity. The inclusion of green spaces and parks in urban planning not only fosters a connection to nature but also offers areas for communal activities.

Concurrently, public health campaigns and educational initiatives are advocating for plant-based nutrition, urging individuals and communities to embrace diets abundant in fruits, vegetables, whole grains, and legumes.

Efforts to establish and endorse community gardens empower residents to cultivate their own fresh produce, nurturing a sense of ownership and connection to food sources. Taking inspiration from the vibrant lifestyles of Blue Zone elders, senior exercise programs are designed to encourage physical activity, balance, and flexibility among older adults. Initiatives promoting intergenerational interactions not only foster social connections but also instil a sense of purpose for both younger and older community members.

Local governments and organisations are enacting programs that actively promote community engagement, the establishment of social support networks, and the creation of communal spaces to facilitate interaction. Initiatives advocating for volunteerism and community service not only offer individuals opportunities to contribute to the well-being of others but also cultivate a profound sense of purpose.

Additionally, educational programs on mindfulness and meditation techniques are being implemented in various settings, aiming to foster stress reduction and enhance mental well-being.

Mental health services, centred on cultivating resilience and coping strategies, find inspiration in the principles of Blue Zones. Corporations are integrating wellness programs into their frameworks, prioritising physical activity, stress management, and a balanced work-life approach, drawing insights from the Blue Zone philosophy. Innovations in workplace policies, including flexible schedules and remote work options, are designed to assist employees in achieving an improved work-life balance.

Culinary programs and workshops are imparting skills to individuals on crafting nutritious and plant-based meals, inspired by the dietary patterns observed in Blue Zones. Efforts promoting the consumption of locally sourced and seasonal foods are fostering sustainable and health-conscious eating habits.

Digital health tools, encompassing apps and wearables, motivate individuals to monitor and enhance their well-being by tracking physical activity, nutrition, and stress levels. The incorporation of telehealth services is enhancing healthcare accessibility, particularly benefiting individuals in remote areas.

Educational programs championing lifelong learning and intellectual stimulation draw inspiration from the Blue Zone's emphasis on sustained mental engagement. Educational institutions are integrating curricula that underscore healthy living, nutrition, and physical activity starting from an early age.

Health advocates and organisations are actively advocating for policy reforms that foster health-promoting environments, including regulations on tobacco, food labelling, and urban planning. The focus of advocacy endeavours is on empowering communities to actively engage in decision-making processes related to health and well-being.